Pathophysiology
of Haemostasis
and Thrombosis

General Information

AF886296

Publication data: 'Pathophysiology of Haemostasis and Thrombosis' is published 6 times a year. Volume 32 with 6 issues appears in 2002.

Subscription rates: Subscriptions run for a full calendar year. Prices are given per volume.
Personal subscription:
Subscription + postage and handling
CHF 439.– + CHF 28.80 Europe
CHF 439.– + CHF 42.70 Overseas
USD 337.50 + USD 28.80
+ online subscription per volume:
CHF 39.– / USD 30.00
(Must be in the name of, billed to, and paid by an individual. Order must be marked 'personal subscription'.)
Institutional subscription:
Subscription + postage and handling
CHF 878.– + CHF 36.– Europe
CHF 878.– + CHF 53.40 Overseas
USD 675.00 + USD 36.00
+ online subscription per volume:
CHF 58.– / USD 45.00
Airmail postage: CHF 36.–, USD 30.00.
(Extra per volume.)
Discount subscription prices:
Gesellschaft für Thrombose- und Haemostase-Forschung;
International Society of Haematology.

Microforms: Please direct all enquiries and orders to:
University Microfilms Inc.
300 North Zeeb Road, P.O. Box 1346
Ann Arbor, MI 48106-1346 (USA)

Subscription orders: Orders can be placed at agencies, bookstores, directly with the
Publisher S. Karger AG, P.O. Box,
CH–4009 Basel (Switzerland)
or with any of the following distributors:
Deutschland: S. Karger GmbH, Postfach
D–79095 Freiburg
France: Librairie Luginbühl
36, bd de Latour-Maubourg
F–75007 Paris
Great Britain, Ireland: S. Karger Publishers
58 Grove Hill Road
Tunbridge Wells, Kent TN1 1SP, UK
USA: S. Karger Publishers, Inc.
26 West Avon Road, P.O. Box 529
Farmington, CT 06085, USA
India, Bangladesh, Sri Lanka:
Panther Publishers Private Ltd.
39, 6th Cross
Wilson Gardens
Bangalore 560 027, India
Japan: Katakura Libri, Inc.
2F, Marushima Bldg, 4-6-17, Yushima,
Bunkyo-ku, Tokyo 113-0034, Japan

Change of address: Both old and new address should be sent to the subscription source.

Single issues and back volumes: Information can be obtained through the Publisher.

Advertising: Correspondence and rate requests should be addressed to the Publisher.

Bibliographic indices: This journal is regularly listed in bibliographic services, including *Medline/PubMed.*

Copying: This journal has been registered with the Copyright Clearance Center (CCC), as indicated by the code appearing on the first page of each article.

For readers in the US, this code signals consent for copying of articles for personal or internal use, or for the personal or internal use of specific clients, provided that the stated fee is paid per copy directly to:
Copyright Clearance Center Inc.
222 Rosewood Drive
Danvers, MA 01923 (USA).
A copy of the first page of the article must accompany payment. Consent does not extend to copying for general distribution, for promotion, for creating new works, or for resale. In these cases, specific written permission must be obtained from the copyright owner,
S. Karger AG, P.O. Box,
CH–4009 Basel (Switzerland).

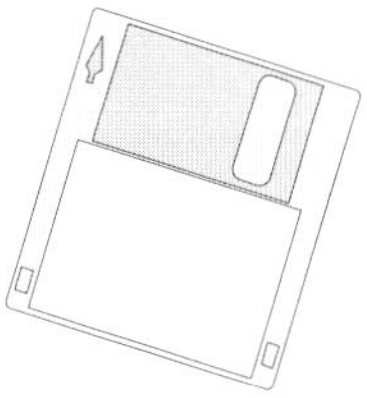

Disk Submission

A **comprehensive version** of these guidelines for the **submission of manuscripts and illustrations on disk** can be accessed online under **www.karger.com/journals/disksub.htm** or requested as a leaflet from the editorial department.

Please follow the general rules on style and arrangement in the **'Guidelines for Authors'** of the journal. Submit a **double-spaced printout** of your manuscript matching the file on disk exactly.

Technical Information
Store only data pertinent to this manuscript. Include your fonts (screen and printer fonts for Macintosh). For a **text only** manuscript, use a 3.5-inch disk. For **text and illustrations,** use 3.5 or 5.25 Magneto Optical Disc; CD-ROM (DOS or hybrid); iomage Zip/DOS (100 MB), or 44 MB, 88 MB or 200 MB SyQuest. Compress extensive data using ZIP format.

Data Description
Label your disk with the **title of the journal or book** for which it is submitted; a **short version** of the paper's title; your **name,** postal and e-mail address, fax and phone number; **hard- and software** used, including the version; and the **complete list of the file names.** File names consist of eight characters before the dot identifying the file and three characters after the dot identifying the application.

Text and Format
The **preferred word-processing package is MS-Word.** Other commonly used PC text programs and ASCII formats are accepted.
Update your data when you revise subsequent to the reviewer's or editor's decision and mark revisions clearly. Manuscripts accepted for publication are subject to **copy editing:** changes and/or questions will be marked in the manuscript, which will be returned to you with your disk and the galley proofs for checking.
Enter your text continuously flush left. Do not use any layout functions. Do not split words at the end of a line. **Do not use indentations.** Use a blank line before and a hard return at the end of paragraphs.
Arrange headings flush left. Insert only **one space after punctuation marks.** Insert Greek letters, mathematical symbols etc. with your word-processing program. Use **boldface and italics** as well as sub- and superscript where appropriate.
Tables are part of the text and should be placed at the end of the text file. Separate the individual parts of a table by lines. Use the tabulator instead of spaces. Format operation data on one line in the same column. **Legends to illustrations are part of the text** and should also be listed at the end of the text file.

Illustrations
Store illustrations as separate files: do not integrate them in your text. Export **line drawings/vector graphics** as TIF, EPS or WMF format. Use Photoshop for processing and retouching **scanned halftone images.** Save the original scan and the processed version. Export **black and white or color images** as TIF or EPS format in their anticipated size in print.
For detailed information on how to submit illustration data on disk please consult the leaflet or **www.karger.com/journals/disksub.htm.**

KI 98 DISK

KARGER

Fax +41 61 306 12 34
E-Mail karger@karger.ch
www.karger.com

The Guidelines for Authors are available at:
www.karger.com/journals/pht

Discusses past experiences with and future roles of this filtration procedure

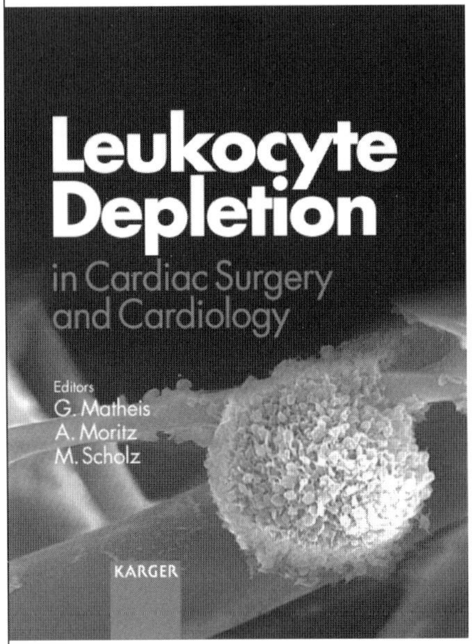

Leukocyte Depletion in Cardiac Surgery and Cardiology

Cardiovascular System; Surgery; Anesthesiology, Transfusion Medicine, Medical Engineering, Immunology

Editors
Georg Matheis
Anton Moritz
Martin Scholz

The concept of leukocyte depletion has been acknowledged as a mandatory procedure in transfusion medicine for a while. Within recent years, leukocyte removal filters have also become a more and more important tool in cardiac surgery, where this procedure is a logical strategy to limit neutrophil-mediated disorders.
The complex biology of neutrophils therefore represents a major point of interest of this volume. Different clinical settings and the corresponding leukocyte filtration methods are a further topic of discussion, including transfusion, transplantation, perfusion and filtration modalities, blood cardioplegia as well as future filtration strategies such as bioactive cytokine filters. Aiming to provide an overview of the experience with experimental and clinical leukocyte filtration and of the state-of-the-art in clinical application, this book also gives an outlook on the possible future role of leukocyte depletion in cardiac surgery and cardiology. It contains information valuable to all perfusionists and clinicians dealing with cardiac surgery and invasive cardiology, and will certainly be read with interest by medical engineers and investigators working in the fields of biotechnology, experimental surgery or cardiology.

KI 02229

Contents

www.karger.com/cardiovascular_system

Leukocyte Depletion in Cardiac Surgery and Cardiology
Editors: Matheis, G.; Moritz, A.; Scholz, M. (Frankfurt)
X + 158 p., 32 fig., 15 tab., hard cover, 2002
CHF 148.– / EUR 105.50 / USD 128.75
Prices subject to change
EUR price for Germany, USD price for USA only
ISBN 3–8055–7281–6

KARGER

Order Form

Please send: ____ copy/ies
Postage and handling free with prepayment

Payment:
☐ Check enclosed ☐ Please bill me

Please charge to my credit card
☐ American Express ☐ Diners ☐ Eurocard
☐ MasterCard ☐ Visa

Card No.: ____________________

Exp. date: ____________________

Orders may be placed with any bookshop, subscription agency, directly with the publisher or through a Karger distributor.

Fax: +41 61 306 12 34
S. Karger AG, P.O. Box, CH–4009 Basel (Switzerland)
E-Mail karger@karger.ch, **www.karger.com**

Name/Address: ____________________

Date: ____________________

Signature: ____________________

32 | S1 | 02
Released April 2002
ISSN 1424–8832
32(suppl 1) 1–54 (2002)

Supplement for subscribers free of charge

Pathophysiology of Haemostasis and Thrombosis

Evidence-Based Haemostasis

Symposium, Dublin, November 9–11, 2001

Guest Editor
Owen P. Smith, Dublin

S. Karger
Medical and Scientific
Publishers
Basel • Freiburg
Paris • London
New York • New Delhi
Bangkok • Singapore
Tokyo • Sydney

KARGER

From epidemiology to pathogenesis and treatment

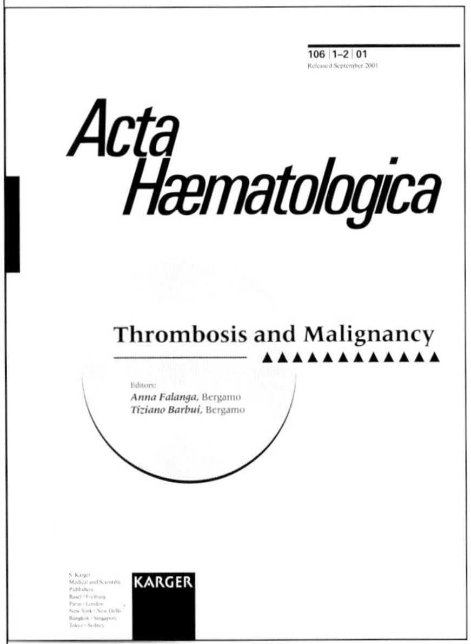

Thrombosis and Malignancy

Editors

Anna Falanga
Tiziano Barbui

Hematology; Oncology

Contents

For over a hundred years, thrombosis has been known to contribute significantly to the morbidity and mortality of malignant disease. In the last decades, major advances in the investigation of the relationship between tumor growth and blood coagulation have been achieved, showing this complex phenomenon to be the second most important cause of death in cancer patients.
This special issue of Acta Haematologica covers the most relevant aspects of thromboembolism in malignancy, from epidemiology to pathogenesis and treatment. All important epidemiological studies are critically reviewed, and it is demonstrated that thrombosis often represents the earliest clinical manifestation of cancer or can be triggered by surgery or other predisposing conditions such as chemotherapy. Further, pathogenetic mechanisms are described, and the plausibility of the association of thrombosis with malignancy on the basis of various known tumor tissue-specific clot-promoting properties is shown. The issue revisits all varieties of clinical pictures associated with malignancy: subclinical hypercoagulable conditions as well as systemic syndromes like disseminated intravascular coagulation, thrombotic microangiopathy, and hepatic veno-occlusive disease. Finally, new concepts for the prophylaxis in surgical or medical conditions are discussed, and suggestions for treating these complications are provided.
'Thrombosis and Malignancy' is a valuable source of information for vascular biologists, physiologists and molecular biologists and other scientists working in the fields of thrombogenesis and tumor progression. But also oncologists, hematologists, internists or surgeons interested in the identification, prevention and treatment of thrombohemorrhagic complications in cancer patients might greatly benefit from this publication.

KI 01265

www.karger.com/journals/aha

Acta Haematologica
Editor: Ben-Bassat, I. (Tel Hashomer)
ISSN 0001–5792
Special issue: Vol. 106, No. 1–2 (2001)
Included in subscription

Thrombosis and Malignancy
Editors: Falanga, A.; Barbui, T. (Bergamo)
88 p., 11 fig., 13 tab., soft cover, 2001
CHF 39.– / EUR 28.– / USD 34.00
Prices subject to change
EUR price for Germany, USD price for USA only
ISBN 3–8055–7305–7

KARGER

Order Form

Please send: ___ copy/ies

Postage and handling free with prepayment

Payment:
☐ Check enclosed ☐ Please bill me

Please charge to my credit card
☐ American Express ☐ Diners ☐ Eurocard
☐ MasterCard ☐ Visa

Card No.: ______

Exp. date: ______

☐ Please send a free sample copy of the journal **Acta Haematologica**

Orders may be placed with any bookshop, subscription agency, directly with the publisher or through a Karger distributor.

Fax: +41 61 306 12 34
S. Karger AG, P.O. Box, CH–4009 Basel (Switzerland)
E-Mail karger@karger.ch, **www.karger.com**

Name/Address: ______

Date: ______

Signature: ______

Official Journal of the 'Mediterranean League against Thromboembolic Diseases'

Pathophysiology of Haemostasis and Thrombosis

KARGER

Printed in Switzerland
on acid-free paper by
Reinhardt Druck, Basel

Appears bimonthly:
1 volume per year
(6 issues)

Guidelines for Authors

Pathophysiology of Haemostasis and Thrombosis

Submission

Only original papers written in English that communicate novel findings in the field of haemostasis and thrombosis are considered. Both contributions to the basic understanding of these processes and reports on clinical management of disorders in this field are acceptable. Manuscripts should be sent to:

Editorial Office
'Pathophysiology of Haemostasis and Thrombosis'
attn. Mrs. T. Camphuisen-Engel
Maastricht University
Department of Biochemistry
Faculty of Medicine II, Level 4
P.O. Box 616
NL–6200 MD Maastricht (The Netherlands)
Tel. +31 43 388 1678/1674
Fax +31 43 388 4159
E-Mail T.Camphuisen@bioch.unimaas.nl

Manuscripts should be submitted in triplicate (with three sets of illustrations of which one is an original), typewritten double-spaced on one side of the paper, with a wide margin.

Conditions

All manuscripts are subject to editorial review. A manuscript is to be considered rejected when an author does not return a revised manuscript within 3 months of receiving the suggestions for revision, unless the author explains further delay. Manuscripts are received with the explicit understanding that they are not under simultaneous consideration by any other publication. Submission of an article for publication implies the transfer of the copyright from the author to the publisher upon acceptance. Accepted papers become the permanent property of 'Pathophysiology of Haemostasis and Thrombosis' and may not be reproduced by any means, in whole or in part, without the written consent of both the author and the publisher. It is the author's responsibility to obtain permission to reproduce illustrations, tables, etc. from other publications.

Arrangement

Title page: The first page of each paper should indicate the title, the authors' names, and the institute where the work was conducted. A short title for use as running head as well as the full address of the author to whom correspondence should be sent are also required.

Full address: The exact postal address complete with postal code must be given at the bottom of the title page. Please also supply phone and fax numbers, as well as your e-mail address.

Key words: For indexing purposes, a list of 3–10 key words in English is essential.

Abstract: Each paper needs an abstract of up to 10 lines.

Small type: Paragraphs which can or must be set in smaller type (case histories, test methods, etc.) should be indicated with a 'p' (petit) in the margin on the left-hand side.

Footnotes: Avoid footnotes. When essential, they are numbered consecutively and typed at the foot of the appropriate page.

Tables and illustrations: Tables and illustrations (both numbered in Arabic numerals) should be prepared on separate sheets. Tables require a heading and figures a legend, also prepared on a separate sheet. For the reproduction of illustrations, only good drawings and original photographs can be accepted; negatives or photocopies cannot be used. Due to technical reasons, figures with a screen background should not be submitted. When possible, group several illustrations on one block for reproduction (max. size 181 × 223 mm) or provide crop marks. On the back of each illustration, indicate its number, the author's name, and 'top' with a soft pencil.

Color illustrations: Up to 6 color illustrations per page can be integrated within the text at the reduced price of CHF 660.– / USD 545.00 per page. Color illustrations are reproduced at the author's expense.

References: In the text identify references by Arabic numerals [in square brackets]. Material submitted for publication but not yet accepted should be noted as 'unpublished data' and not be included in the reference list. The list of references should include only those publications which are cited in the text. Do not alphabetize; number references in the order in which they are first mentioned in the text. The surnames of the authors followed by initials should be given. There should be no punctuation other than a comma to separate the authors. Cite all authors, 'et al' is not sufficient. Abbreviate journal names according to the Index Medicus system. (Also see International Committee of Medical Journal Editors: Uniform requirements for manuscripts submitted to biomedical journals. N Engl J Med 1997;336:309–315.)

(a) Papers published in periodicals: Sun J, Koto H, Chung KF: Interaction of ozone and allergen challenges on bronchial responsiveness and inflammation in sensitised guinea pigs. Int Arch Allergy Immunol 1997;112:191–195.
(b) Monographs: Matthews DE, Farewell VT: Using and Understanding Medical Statistics, ed 3, revised. Basel, Karger, 1996.
(c) Edited books: Parren PWHI, Burton DR: Antibodies against HIV-1 from phage display libraries: Mapping of an immune response and progress towards antiviral immunotherapy; in Capra JD (ed): Antibody Engineering. Chem Immunol. Basel, Karger, 1997, vol 65, pp 18–56.

Page charges

There are no page charges for papers of 4 or fewer printed pages (including tables, illustrations and references). Each additional complete or partial page is charged to the author at CHF 275.– / USD 196.00. The allotted size of a paper is equal to approx. 12 manuscript pages (including tables, illustrations and references).

Galley proofs

Unless indicated otherwise, galley proofs are sent to the first-named author and should be returned with the least possible delay. Alterations made in galley proofs, other than the correction of printer's errors, are charged to the author. No page proofs are supplied.

Reprints

Order forms and a price list are sent with the galley proofs. Orders submitted after the issue is printed are subject to considerably higher prices.

KARGER

Fax + 41 61 306 12 34
E-Mail karger@karger.ch
www.karger.com

The Guidelines for Authors are available at:
www.karger.com/journals/pht/pht_gl.htm

Pathophysiology
of Haemostasis
and Thrombosis

Evidence-Based Haemostasis

Symposium, Dublin, November 9–11, 2001

Guest Editor
Owen P. Smith, Dublin

12 figures and 11 tables, 2002

KARGER

Basel · Freiburg · Paris · London · New York ·
New Delhi · Bangkok · Singapore · Tokyo · Sydney

The symposium and the publication of this supplement were supported by an educational grant from Haematology Business Unit, Novo Nordisk.

S. Karger
Medical and Scientific Publishers
Basel · Freiburg · Paris · London
New York · New Delhi · Bangkok
Singapore · Tokyo · Sydney

Drug Dosage
The authors and the publisher have exerted every effort to ensure that drug selection and dosage set forth in this text are in accord with current recommendations and practice at the time of publication. However, in view of ongoing research, changes in government regulations, and the constant flow of information relating to drug therapy and drug reactions, the reader is urged to check the package insert for each drug for any change in indications and dosage and for added warnings and precautions. This is particularly important when the recommended agent is a new and/or infrequently employed drug.

Printed in Switzerland on acid-free paper by
Reinhardt Druck, Basel
ISBN 3–8055–7418–5

KARGER

Fax + 41 61 306 12 34
E-Mail karger@karger.ch
www.karger.com

Vol. 32, Suppl. 1, 2002

Pathophysiology of Haemostasis and Thrombosis

Contents

KARGER

Fax + 41 61 306 12 34
E-Mail karger@karger.ch
www.karger.com

Access to full text and tables of contents, including tentative ones for forthcoming issues:
www.karger.com/journals/pht/pht_bk.htm

Pathophysiology of Haemostasis and Thrombosis

Preface

Evidence-based medicine is defined as the conscientious, explicit and judicious use of current best evidence in making decisions about the care of individual patients (Sackett et al, McMaster University, 1991). The symposium 'Evidence based haemostasis', held in Dublin on November 9–10, 2001, provided a landmark forum for the presentation of latest best evidence to haematologists concerned with achieving haemostasis in both haemophiliac and non-haemophiliac patients.

The primary function of this meeting was to address the needs of the practising haematologist/coagulation specialist with respect to determining the benefits and risks (if any) of recombinant activated factor VII (rFVIIa; NovoSeven®) compared with alternative patient management strategies.

Almost 205,000 standard dosages of rFVIIa have been given to patients since it became available over a decade ago, but publications relating to its use remain relatively sparse. The data presented at the Dublin symposium clarified issues relating to the efficacy of this life-saving agent. It is clear that rFVIIa has revolutionised the treatment of haemophiliac patients with inhibitors to coagulation therapy, a problem which affects a small but significant proportion of haemophiliacs.

The initial sessions of the symposium included reviews of the evidence for the use of rFVIIa and the alternatives – porcine factor VIII and activated prothrombin complex concentrates – in patients with haemophilia and inhibitors comparing the data for the different treatment options, it is clear that rFVIIa is associated with an extremely high response rate. In addition, excellent results have been obtained from the use of rFVIIa in children with haemophilia and high responding inhibitors. Recombinant FVIIa provides vital cover for such patients until immune tolerance therapy (ITT) becomes effective and also allows the insertion of a central venous catheter to facilitate ITT.

Cost

A major concern over the use of rFVIIa has been the cost of this expensive-to-produce treatment. However, economic analyses presented at the symposium showed convincingly that treatment with rFVIIa can be cheaper than the alternatives such as FEIBA. This is because the good efficacy of rFVIIa means that less treatment is needed in order to achieve successful results.

Further Indications

Recombinant FVIIa holds promise in several indications beyond inhibitor patients, for example in other situations involving impaired thrombin generation and in the management of platelet disorders.

KARGER
Fax + 41 61 306 12 34
E-Mail karger@karger.ch
www.karger.com

Accessible online at:
www.karger.com/journals/pht

Intense interest is also mounting in the use of rFVIIa outside the field of coagulopathies, in particular in major bleeding associated with surgery or trauma. As experience increases, rFVIIa is emerging as a treatment which produces almost instant results, often when all other options have failed. Such findings were reported at the meeting from case studies of uncontrolled bleeding in cardiac surgery and in other surgical and trauma situations among patients without existing coagulopathy. These patients showed a rapid and significant reduction in post operative blood loss.

Further ongoing and planned randomised studies may support the use of rFVIIa in general haemostasis management. Planned trials include studies that will address key questions in areas of internal medicine that have major problematical scenarios including orthotopic liver transplantation and stem cell transplantation, as well as further studies of cardiac surgery in children and adults.

The Future

In the opening session of this symposium, Dr. William Murphy outlined how therapeutic options for maintaining haemostasis have evolved to minimise disease transmission associated with the use of blood products. Recombinant products have arisen as awareness has grown of the risks from blood products and the desire to avoid allogeneic blood. This symposium has confirmed that rFVIIa has a huge potential in reducing the amount of exposure to allogeneic blood, and over time it is likely to displace plasma derived bypassing agents throughout the western world.

Not only does rFVIIa have a strong foothold in haemophilia management, but we are also entering an era of recombinant coagulation therapeutics in intensive care of patients without coagulopathies. At the same time as gaining a wealth of clinical experience in the use of rFVIIa, we are also learning much more about how this agent works. Hence as the evidence base expands, clinical decisions to use rFVIIa can be made with increasing confidence.

Owen P. Smith

Pathophysiology of Haemostasis and Thrombosis

Pathophysiol Haemost Thromb 2002;32(suppl 1):1–4

Disease Transmission by Blood Products: Past, Present and Future

William G. Murphy

Irish Blood Transfusion Service, Dublin, Ireland

Key Words
Blood products · Safety · Infection · Non-linear systems

Abstract
Transfusion of blood and blood products has been associated with transmission of infectious agents. However, it is probable that blood products are currently very safe and that pooled virus-inactivated products from remunerated donors are now safer than untreated single voluntary donor components. Although the transmission events of the past and the present are reasonably well understood, reliance on a linear approach to predict safety in the future is open to criticism. Indeed, it was not possible to predict the extent or consequences of the AIDS epidemic or of hepatitis C transmission. Moreover, although variant Creutzfeldt-Jakob disease (vCJD) may not be transmitted to any large extent by transfusion of manufactured blood products, this will be due more to good fortune than good judgement – this agent could have escaped the screening, testing and eradication methods on which current confidence in blood product safety depends. Similarly, the emergence of a highly resistant non-enveloped virus, or even of another previously unrecognised disease-causing agent, could result in new threats from transfusion of blood components and products. The ecology of blood transfusion is exquisitely sensitive to variations in starting conditions, a situation typical of a chaotic rather than a linear system. Seemingly trivial events, often apparently unrelated to blood transfusion, have had enormous consequences in this field. Whatever the events that introduced simian immunodeficiency virus to humans or scrapie to cattle, they were a long way from those involved in the manufacture of blood products. In such a setting, reliance on methods that deal effectively with known threats (such as encapsulated viruses and bacteria) without adequate investigation and management of the intrinsic sensitivity to unpredictable events, leaves open the possibility of further infections emerging in the future. It is this reality that will ultimately result in the eradication of the transfusion of donor-derived blood and blood products in the developed world. In addition, all infections with a long disease-free incubation period in the host that can be transmitted in blood will eventually be over-expressed in groups that are exposed to blood either recreationally or professionally. As in the past, this could have occurred before testing or decontamination processes have been developed for emerging pathogens. Failure to be able to rely on completely risk-free donors, in both the voluntary and non-voluntary sides of the blood industry, continues to offer the potential for the transmission of infectious diseases in the future.

KARGER
Fax +41 61 306 12 34
E-Mail karger@karger.ch
www.karger.com

1424–8832/02/0327–0001$18.50/0

Accessible online at:
www.karger.com/journals/pht

Dr. William Murphy
Irish Blood Transfusion Service, James's Street
Dublin 8 (Ireland)
Tel. +353 1432 2800, Fax +353 1432 2931
E-Mail Tess.Maguire@ibts.ie

Introduction

Evidence-based medicine uses data from the past and present to make predictions with a greater or lesser degree of confidence about the future. In the case of blood and blood product safety, the value of such predictions requires careful assessment and considerable scepticism. Although considerable effort has gone into making blood products as safe as possible, their future safety depends on many more variables than are immediately obvious. The screening techniques that have been developed so far can only work against diseases that have already been identified. Inactivation techniques are similarly limited, and are not universally effective. Further, as yet unrecognisable risks may exist, making it impossible to make assertions of the safety of the blood supply based on what we currently know. Science does not predict the future, and may be 'nothing more than a sharper set of questions to guide us through the fog' [1] – we cannot make assertions or predictions of future events, and, if we persist in doing so we may impede appropriate planning based on realistic uncertainty.

Past Infections in Blood Products

The ecology of blood collection, storage and transfusion generates distinct patterns of disease. The use of fresh unstored blood and vein-to-vein transfusion resulted in syphilis being a major concern in the early years of blood transfusion. Storage of blood in the cold in turn led to the emergence of psychrophilic bacteria as a lethal complication in the 1940s and 1950s. In the 1970s the widespread acceptance of 22°C as the optimum temperature for platelet storage was accompanied by the rise of serious gram-positive and gram-negative infections from transfusion of these components.

Current Infections

Malaria, parvovirus B19, and cytomegalovirus are still major infectious problems from blood transfusion, although the extent is not well documented globally. These infections are not routinely screened for in all donations. While there remains a small risk of undetected window period infections from HIV and hepatitis C in developed countries, these agents can be expected to be removed from blood derivatives during manufacture. This has led to the current situation where pooled virus inactivated derivatives are considered safer than non-pooled single-donor non-virus inactivated products, at least in so far as such agents are concerned.

However, current inactivation techniques applied to blood derivatives do not remove all infectious agents. TT virus, while it may not be associated with transmissible morbidity, nevertheless serves as a marker for viral resilience to current inactivation techniques. A recent study showed that this virus could be transmitted via the albumin used in the manufacture of recombinant VIIIc and IX [2]. Similarly, parvovirus B19 can escape eradication in the manufacturing of albumin, indicating that the potential exists for viral transmission from future blood products [3].

Future Infections

Non-Linear Science and Blood Transfusion

While formal proof is lacking, the blood transfusion ecosystem shows some characteristics of the chaotic behaviour found in systems composed of complex interdependent components. For example, a seemingly trivial or remote event in the system can result in catastrophic consequences over considerable ranges of space and time.

HIV

An example of a minor, apparently unrelated change with disastrous consequences was the appearance of HIV in blood transfusion in the 1980s. It is possible that the transmission of simian immunodeficiency virus to humans may have been occurring in West Africa for a long time previously, but it was the beginning of forest clearance in the area that allowed the infection to spread out of the forest to the general population. Thus an apparently unrelated commercial desire for hardwoods may have led to thousands of deaths from transfusion and millions of deaths from AIDS, and will probably lead to collapse of national economies.

Yersinia Infection

A less dramatic but nonetheless intriguing example of a minor event having a major impact could have been the emergence of *Y. enterocolitica* as a hazard of transfusion in 1978. This organism, which carries a 70% mortality as a septic complication of blood transfusion, was not previously associated with blood transfusion, and it is unlikely that it would have been missed as a diagnosis. There have been well over 100 cases since, emerging in blood transfusion recipients in several countries around the same time. However, there seems to have been no significant change in epidemiology in the general population. The outbreak followed the introduction of plasma reduction during the late 1970s, and all cases were from plasma-reduced blood units, although the relationship is not clear. Normally, pathogenic Yersinia are killed as blood cools from between 32 and 10°C [4]. Plasma reduction shortens the time for blood cooling, and this may have affected the susceptibility of the organism to complement killing.

However, it is also very possible that plasma reduction had an unexpected benefit, preventing thousands of deaths from fluid overload.

Classic linear approaches will not provide definitive answers to the appearance of Yersinia in blood transfusion. Similarly, such approaches will not explain and did not predict a surge in maternal deaths from haemorrhage between 1988 and 1990 (table 1) [5]. This may have been linked to a rise in the use of red cell concentrates around that time for transfusion in these women rather than whole blood. While this will always remain speculative, it underlines the susceptibility of the blood transfusion world to unexpected events arising from seemingly unrelated triggering factors.

If the blood transfusion system does follow the rules of chaos theory and is therefore a complex non linear system, then it poses a major problem for manipulating the risk of future transmissible infections. Although we have safer blood products now than ever before, the safety precautions can only reliably ward off known threats. Any new, previously uncharacterised infections could emerge unchallenged because current procedures do not test for them or may not inactivate them. For this reason, the use of blood products will remain inherently unsafe. If, for example, variant CJD is not being transmitted by blood products, this is due to luck rather than safety procedures – this agent could have escaped the screening, testing and eradication methods currently in use.

Strategies for Risk Reduction

The future to combating transfusible diseases in a system that, while not utterly unpredictable, is nonetheless subject to the laws of chaos rather than linear science is not totally bleak. Risk reduction in a non-linear system is not a simple affair, but recognition of the chaotic nature of the problem will be of some use, not least if it avoids spurious reliance on assertions based on an invalid linear approach. 'Not only in research, but in the everyday world of politics and economics, we would all be better off if more people realised that simple non-linear systems do not necessarily possess simple dynamical properties' [6].

Table 1. Maternal deaths from haemorrhage in the UK, 1985–1993, showing an as yet unexplained rise in deaths between1988–1990

Number of maternal deaths from haemorrhage	10	22	12
Time period	85–87	81–90	91–93

Approaches to risk reduction in complex systems might include removal of feedback lops where possible, which should have the effect of reducing the rate of generation of unpredictable effects. This approach provides a rational basis for the removal of paid donors, and for the removal of transfused donors, as sources of blood and plasma. While such donors may not provide a current source of infection, they do provide an important feedback loop that increases the variability of the system.

Paid Donations as a Feedback Loop

Infections (other than bacterial contamination) transmissible by blood products have several more or less essential characteristics: they are spread by blood contact such as needle-sharing in IV drug abusers; they do not result in clinical disease until some time after infectivity in the host is established, and a test for infectivity in donors is not available until the existence of the disease is established. This set of preconditions has resulted in the fact that any new infection transmitted by blood transfusion will be over-represented in professional blood and plasma donors by the time screening is put in place and subject to exponential spread within this group.

This was true for HIV, hepatitis B and hepatitis C [7]. It is also true for HCV NAT screening – data from Germany indicate that hepatitis C positivity by NAT testing is eight times more likely from paid rather than non-remunerated donors (17 positive donors out of 2.3 million donations in paid donors versus 11 out of 12.7 million non-remunerated donors – relative risk 8.394 (95% CI 3.9–17.9) $p < 0.0001$) [8]. It is evident that paid donors are withholding information on risk activity at a much higher rate than non-remunerated donors.

While previously transfused individuals represent a lesser risk, they do provide a feedback loop that amplifies any infection that is dormant, unscreened for, and not removed during processing and manufacture.

Ultimately this complex and largely unpredictable behaviour in the transfusion ecosystem will only be controlled by abandoning the use of blood and blood products. While this in itself would give rise to unpredictable effects elsewhere in the universe of healthcare, it is extremely important that unfounded reassurances on blood safety do not obstruct proper planning for future safety.

Conclusion

Current confidence in the safety of blood and blood products is misguided. Our methods of screening and inactivation of viruses are simply linear solutions which will not work on sufficiently large scales of time and space for a non-linear complex system such as blood transfusion. Hence it would be inappropriate to take comfort from the successful control of HCV, HIV, and other currently recognised infections. We have not yet developed the tools in the blood product industry or in public health to predict and then cope with new risks as they arise. The system is extremely sensitive to unpredictable events, leaving it highly vulnerable to future threats. Further disastrous epidemics could well arise in the future.

It is this unpredictability that will eventually lead to the eradication of the transfusion of donor-derived blood and blood products.

References

1 May R: Risk and Uncertainty. Nature 2001; 411:891.
2 Azzi A, Santis R, Morfini M, Zakrzewska K, Musso R, Santagostino E, Castarnan G: TT virus contaminates first-generation recombinant factor VII concentrates. Blood 2001;98: 2571–2573.
3 Saldanha J, Minor P: Detection of human parvovirus B19 DNA in plasma pools and blood products derived from these pools: Implications for efficacy and consistency of removal of B19 DNA during manufacture. Br J Haematol 1996;93:714–719.
4 Gibb AP, Martin KM, Davidson GA, Walker B, Murphy WG: Modelling the growth of Yersinia enterocolitica in donated blood. Transfusion 1994;34:304–310.
5 Department of Health: Why Mothers Die: Report on Confidential Enquiries into Maternal Deaths 1994/96. London: Her Majesty's Stationery Office, 1998.
6 May R: Simple mathematical models with very complicated dynamics. Nature 1976;261:459–467.
7 Eastlund T: Monetary blood donation incentives and the risk of transfusion-transmitted infection. Transfusion 1998;38:874–882.
8 Seifried E, Hitzler W: Status of NAT screening for HCV, HIV and HBV: Experience in Germany. Infus Ther Transfusion Medicine 2001; 28:231 (abstract).

Pathophysiology of Haemostasis and Thrombosis

Pathophysiol Haemost Thromb 2002;32(suppl 1):5–8

The Evidence behind Inhibitor Treatment with Porcine Factor VIII

Christine A. Lee

The Haemophilia Centre and Haemostasis Unit, Royal Free Hospital NHS Trust, London, UK

Key Words

Porcine FVIII · Inhibitor · Pharmacokinetics · Hybrid FVIII · Acquired

Abstract

Factor VIII auto- and alloantibodies neutralise porcine factor VIII to a lesser extent than factor VIII of human origin. The reduced reactivity of the porcine molecule, predominantly due to sequence variation in the A2 and C2 domains, has been the rationale for using porcine factor VIII to secure haemostasis for patients with factor VIII inhibitors. Porcine factor VIII has been shown to provide effective haemostatic control particularly for patients with intermediate inhibitor titres with limited porcine cross-reactivity. Small studies have indicated porcine factor VIII can be associated with desensitisation of some factor VIII inhibitor patients. Porcine factor VIII has been shown to produce mild platelet agglutination, an effect that may enhance its efficacy. Adverse reactions are dose-related and do not preclude safe and effective long-term home use for the subgroup of inhibitor patients with modest or absent anamnestic response. Efforts to secure source plasma free of viral markers, particularly porcine parvovirus, have limited the supply of this therapeutic product.

Introduction

Porcine factor (F)VIII (Hyate:C®) is a second-generation FVIII concentrate of porcine plasma origin, fractionated using a polyelectrolyte resin. Although there is no specific viral attenuation step during the production of this concentrate, a four-cell line general viral screen and a polymerase chain reaction source plasma screen for porcine parvovirus are performed. Porcine FVIII has not been shown to transmit viral disease.

The first published clinical experience with polyelectrolyte fractionated porcine FVIII concentrate in the treatment of haemophilic patients with antibodies to FVIII was reported in 1984 [1]. It is of interest that the first patient to be treated in 1980 is still using this treatment as home therapy. This review will present the published evidence base for the clinical use of porcine FVIII, together with a brief summary of research development of porcine-human FVIII hybrid constructs.

Porcine FVIII as an Inhibitor Bypassing Agent

Porcine FVIII has been effective in treating acute bleeding in patients with congenital or acquired haemophilia. The first publication gave a detailed description of 45 treatment courses in eight inhibitor patients, a total of 297 infusions [1]. Where no cross-reactivity to porcine

KARGER
Fax +41 61 306 12 34
E-Mail karger@karger.ch
www.karger.com

1424–8832/02/0327–0005$18.50/0

Accessible online at:
www.karger.com/journals/pht

Prof. Christine Lee, Centre Director
Royal Free Hospital, Pond Street
London, NW3 2QG (UK)
Tel. +44 207 7830 2238, Fax +44 207 7830 2468, E-Mail christine.lee@rfh.nthames.nhs.uk

FVIII was detectable, the mean increment in plasma FVIII was 1.29 IU/dl per IU/kg of porcine factor VIII administered. With increasing porcine FVIII cross-reactivity, factor VIII recovery progressively declined. Where post-infusion FVIII recovery was detectable, clinical response was good and conventional FVIII:C assay could be used to guide dosage. The study concluded that the product was an effective haemostatic agent for patients with FVIII inhibitors, particularly those with intermediate level anti-human FVIII titres where cross-reactivity to porcine FVIII was limited. A study from the United States described 45 life or limb threatening bleeding episodes in 38 patients with high-responding inhibitors [2]. A total of 437 infusions were administered, with a good or excellent response recorded in 71% of bleeds. Adverse reactions occurred in 17 treatment episodes, and responded to antihistamines with or without hydrocortisone. The most common infused dose was 50 IU/kg.

Porcine FVIII concentrate has an advantage over human-derived FVIII in patients with congenital haemophilia and inhibitors since the antibodies have a median of only 15% cross-reactivity with porcine FVIII [3]. In addition, patients with acquired haemophilia usually respond well to porcine FVIII, particularly when they have low or absent anti-porcine inhibitor titres. In general, patients with inhibitor titres of <20 BU/ml have a better response rate than those with higher titres [1]. Some patients with congenital haemophilia maintain low anti-porcine inhibitor titres over long term use and can therefore be treated routinely at home over many years. It is possible that the platelet agglutinating effect of porcine von Willebrand factor (vWF) may contribute to the response in patients with high titre inhibitors. An anamnestic response has been reported to occur in 25–35% of treatments with porcine FVIII, but this risk is relatively low among patients with acquired haemophilia. Most patients with congenital haemophilia can be treated for serious bleeding before the development of clinically significant anti-porcine antibodies.

Home Therapy with Porcine FVIII

Porcine FVIII has been used safely and effectively in the home therapy setting for extended periods. An observational study described the experience of five haemophilia A patients with high-titre, high-responding FVIII alloantibodies who received porcine FVIII for periods of up to 8.5 years [4]. Specific anti-porcine activity developed in all cases, but was generally transient, with only one patient becoming refractory. Of particular interest, all patients lost their anti-human FVIII activity over time. In three cases, human FVIII was re-introduced successfully, with no recurrence of anti-human FVIII activity over 2–3 years of continued therapy. There were no significant transfusion reactions.

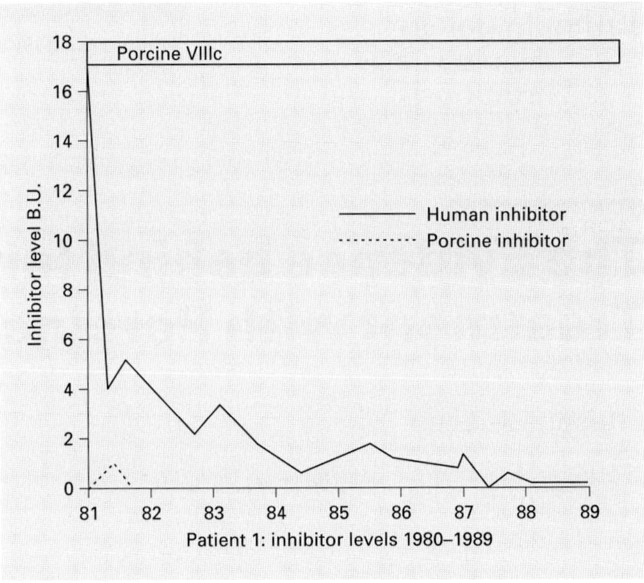

Fig. 1. FVIII desensitisation: inhibitor titres between 1980 and 1989. (From Hay et al, 1997, with permission.)

One of the first inhibitor patients to receive porcine FVIII has used the product as required to treat bleeding episodes for over 20 years. In this time, he has undergone five operative procedures, including total knee arthroplasty, using porcine FVIII for haemostatic control. Figure 1 shows his inhibitor titre declining over time and eventually completely disappearing. A notable feature about this patient is that he never developed a significant cross-reactivity to porcine FVIII [5].

An international survey assessed the side effect profile and use of porcine FVIII for regular or home therapy [3]. The study described 154 inhibitor patients who had used over 15 million IU. The median pre-treatment cross reactivity to the porcine FVIII was 15%. There was no evidence of cross reactivity to the porcine product in 27% of the cases. Figure 2 shows the pre-treatment inhibitor cross reactivity in 137 of the patients. There were very few that had a high cross reactivity and most either had a low cross reactivity or no cross reactivity. Anamnesis was evaluable in 65 patients. Brisk anamnesis, defined as at least a threefold rise in antibody titre following the first treatment,

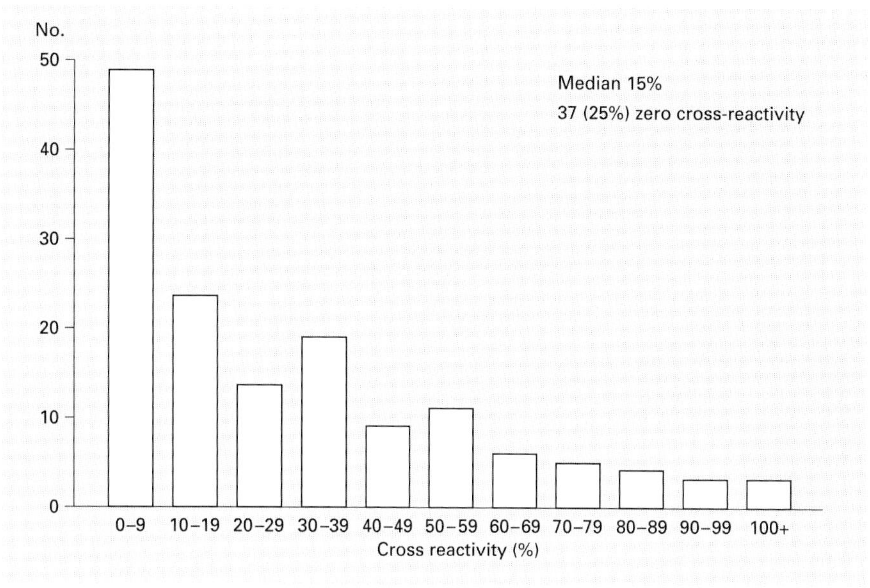

Fig. 2. Histogram of pre-treatment inhibitor cross-reactivity to porcine FVIII:C in 147 patients. (From Hay et al, 1996, with permission.)

occurred in 31% of patients. Importantly, 29% of patients had no anamnestic response following their first treatment and 38% had no such response following multiple treatments. Transfusion reactions occurred after 0.001% of home infusions and in 2.3% of unselected inpatient infusions, with incidence of adverse reactions showing a positive association with dosage.

A post-infusion fall in platelet count is common after administration of porcine FVIII and is due to reversible agglutination by porcine von Willebrand factor. The international survey collected platelet count data around 175 porcine FVIII infusions for 57 individuals. After a median porcine FVIII dose of 96 U/kg, the median fall in platelet count was 34 $\times$ 10^9/l, occurring at about 30 minutes after the infusion. The platelet count reduction was clinically insignificant in all cases [3].

A survey of acquired haemophilia in Europe and the US assessed 74 bleeding episodes in 65 patients [6]. At presentation the median inhibitor titre against human FVIII was 38 BU/ml and against porcine FVIII was 1 BU/ml. The average initial dose of porcine FVIII was 84 IU/kg resulting in a mean increase in plasma FVIII:C of 0.85 IU/ml. Haemostatic response was rated as good or excellent in 78% of cases. The mean duration of therapy was 8.5 days, sufficient in most cases to control bleeding episodes whilst the immune suppression therapy was taking effect.

The half-life of porcine FVIII has considerable inter-individual variability and has been reported to range from 8 to 24 hours. In addition, FVIII levels measured using the chromogenic assay are on average 50% lower than those measured by the one-stage method [7]. The mechanism for this observation has not been clarified. Vial potency of porcine FVIII is assigned by the chromogenic method.

Human/Porcine Hybrid FVIII

Inhibitory antibodies are directed mainly at epitopes in the A2 (residues 373–740), C2 (residues 2173–2332) or A3 domains of the factor VIII molecule. There is evidence that antibodies that recognise epitopes in the A2 domain bind the tenase complex and thereby prevent activation of FX [8]. Antibodies binding to the C2 domain block the interaction of FVIII with phospholipid and may also impair FVIII binding of vWF [9]. Antibodies recognising the A3 domain may inhibit the FVIIIa-FIXa interaction. Recently, recombinant human-porcine hybrid FVIII constructs have been developed with porcine substitutions of the sectors of the human A2 and C2 domains that are known to be more immunogenic [10]. The resultant hybrid human/porcine FVIII molecules have been shown to produce full procoagulant activity, with reduced recognition by neutralising factor VIII antibodies. These constructs may not only be useful as treatment of bleeding in inhibitor patients but may also be less immunogenic than wild-type FVIII for normal use.

Summary

There is a strong evidence base for the use of porcine FVIII, in both congenital haemophilia with FVIII alloantibodies and in acquired haemophilia. It is effective in the subset of inhibitor patients who demonstrate low porcine cross-reactivity. In this group, modest doses – in the region of 30–40 IU/kg – have been used to effectively control bleeding for long term use in the home environment. There are examples where induction of immune tolerance to human FVIII has occurred with long-term use of the porcine product. The prime issue restricting supply of porcine FVIII is the number of pigs infected with porcine parvovirus. While there is no evidence to suggest porcine parvovirus is pathogenic to humans, any infected porcine plasma pools are rejected. This has resulted in rejection of positive pools in 50–80% of cases and has led to extreme shortages in supply of useable plasma.

References

1 Kernoff PB, Thomas ND, Lilley PA, Matthews KB, Goldman E, Tuddenham EG: Clinical experience with polyelectrolyte-fractionated porcine factor VIII concentrate in the treatment of hemophiliacs with antibodies to factor VIII. Blood 1984;663:31–41.

2 Brettler DB, Forsberg AD, Levine PH, Aledort LM, Hilgartner MW, Kasper CK, Lusher JM, McMillan C, Roberts H: The use of porcine factor VIII concentrate (Hyate:C) in the treatment of patients with inhibitor antibodies to factor VIII. A multicenter US experience. Arch Intern Med 1989;149:1381–1385.

3 Hay CR, Lozier JN, Lee CA, Laffan M, Tradati F, Santagostino E, Ciavarella N, Schiavoni M, Fukui H, Yoshioka A, Tietel J, Mannucci PM, Kasper CK: Safety profile of porcine factor VIII and its use as hospital and home-therapy for patients with haemophilia A and inhibitors: The results of an international survey. Thromb Haemost 1996;75:25–29.

4 Hay CR, Laurian Y, Verroust F, Preston FE, Kernoff PB: Induction of immune tolerance in patients with hemophilia A and inhibitors treated with porcine VIIIC by home therapy. Blood 1990;76:882–886.

5 Vyas P, Pasi KJ, Lee CA: Successful long-term treatment with porcine factor VIII of a patient with haemophilia A and an inhibitor to factor VIII. Haemophilia 1996;2:240–243.

6 Morrison AE, Ludlam CA, Kessler C: Use of porcine factor VIII in the treatment of patients with acquired hemophilia. Blood 1993;81:1513–1520.

7 Hermans C, Owens D, Longo G, Morfini M, Lee C.A: Single-dose pharmacokinetics of porcine factor VIII (Hyate C). Thromb Haemost 2002;87:352–353.

8 Lollar P, Parker ET, Curtis JE, Helgerson SL, Hoyer LW, Scott ME, Scandella D: Inhibition of human factor VIIIa by anti-A2 subunit antibodies. J Clin Invest 1994;93:2497–2504.

9 Arai, M, Scandella D, Hoyer LW: Molecular basis of factor VIII inhibition by human antibodies. Antibodies that bind to the factor VIII light chain prevent the interaction of factor VIII with phospholipid. J Clin Invest 1989;83:1978–1984.

10 Lollar P: Analysis of factor VIII inhibitors using hybrid human/porcine factor VIII. Thromb Haemost 1997;78:647–651.

11 Hay CRM, DiMichele D, Rivard G, Rubinger M, Gribble J: Workshop III – porcine factor VIII – continuous infusion, immune tolerance induction and prophylaxis. Haemophilia 1997;3(suppl 3):24–30.

Pathophysiology of Haemostasis and Thrombosis

Pathophysiol Haemost Thromb 2002;32(suppl 1):9–12

Evidence for the Use of Activated Prothrombin Complex Concentrates (aPCCs) in the Treatment of Patients with Haemophilia and Inhibitors

J.T. Wilde

West Midlands Adult Comprehensive Care Haemophilia Centre, University Hospital Birmingham NHS Trust, Birmingham, UK

Key Words
Autoplex®T · FEIBA™ · Inhibitor · aPCC · Bypassing agent

Abstract
FEIBA™ and Autoplex®T have been used to control bleeding in patients with factor VIII or IX inhibitors for over 25 years. The major components of FEIBA™ are thought to be activated factor X and prothrombin, whereas the main active components in Autoplex®T are thought to be activated factors IX and VII. Both products have been found to effectively control approximately 80% of bleeds involving joints and soft tissues. Published experience of their use in surgery is limited. Thrombotic complications have been reported with high dose FEIBA™ therapy and have led to maximum dosage guidelines for this product.

Introduction

The introduction 25 years ago of the activated prothrombin complex concentrates (aPCCs) FEIBA™ (Factor Eight Inhibitor Bypassing Activity concentrate) and Autoplex®T brought about a considerable improvement in the management of patients with haemophilia A or B with inhibitors. These products soon became established as standard first-line treatment for bleeding episodes in this patient group. Both concentrates are produced by in vitro modification of plasma-derived PCCs, resulting in a degree of activation of some of the clotting factors. However, the precise mechanism of action of these aPCCs remains unknown. The aim of this review is to present published experience on the use of aPCCs to control or prevent haemorrhage in patients with neutralising inhibitors to factor VIII or IX, including experience with the specific problems of surgery and dental extractions.

Constituents of FEIBA™ and Autoplex®T

Turecek et al [1] have determined the constituents of FEIBA™. The concentrate contains prothrombin, factors (F) VII, IX and X, activated FVII and FX, thrombin and protein C. Using a rabbit inhibitor model, FEIBA™ triggered coagulation similar to that induced by an enzyme substrate complex of FXa and prothrombin. It has therefore been postulated that when FEIBA™ is introduced, activated FX binds to the phospholipid surface of acti-

KARGER
Fax +41 61 306 12 34
E-Mail karger@karger.ch
www.karger.com

1424–8832/02/0327–0009$18.50/0

Accessible online at:
www.karger.com/journals/pht

Dr. Jonathan T. Wilde, Centre Director
West Midlands Adult Comprehensive Care Haemophilia Centre
Queen Elizabeth Hospital, Edgbaston, Birmingham, B15 2TH (UK)
Tel. +44 121 472 1311 (ext. 3141) Fax +44 121 414 1041, Mobile +44 7831 778309
E-Mail jonathan.wilde@university-b.wmids.nhs.uk

Table 1. Reports of FEIBA efficacy for treatment of inhibitor patients with spontaneous bleeding events

Study	FEIBA dose	Patients	Bleeding episodes	Efficacy
Sjamsoedin [1981]	88 U/kg	15	150	64% (24 h)
Hilgartner [1983]	50–70 U/kg 12 hourly	49	165	91% (72 h)
Hilgartner [1990]	50–75 U/kg 12 hourly	41	106	79% (36 h)
Negrier [1997]	65–100 U/kg 6–12 hourly	60	433	81% (up to 3 doses)

vated platelets at the site of bleeding. Prothrombin is incorporated and the activated FX converts transfused and endogenous prothrombin directly into thrombin, bypassing the need for FVIII and FIX.

Following a detailed analysis of 10 separate batches of Autoplex®T using chromogenic active site-specific immuno assay (CASSIA) technology [2] it has been proposed that this product may work in quite a different way. The CASSIA technique enables the direct specific quantitation of the activated forms of individual clotting factors. High but quite variable concentrations of activated FVII and activated FIX were present within Autoplex®T. Smaller concentrations of activated FX, and negligible concentrations of activated FXI and thrombin were also found. The concentrations of activated FVII were considered not sufficient to directly activate significant amounts of FX. The authors proposed that the activated FIX was in sufficient concentrations to be incorporated on to phospholipid membranes causing activation of endogenous FVII. This coupled with the activated FVII in the concentrate were considered sufficient to enable direct FX activation in large enough quantities to bypass the need for endogenous FVIII and FIX.

Clinical Efficacy

FEIBA™ and Autoplex®T have been reported to have similar clinical efficacy, controlling approximately 80% of spontaneous joint and soft tissue bleeds in inhibitor patients.

Table 1 summarises the major trials assessing the clinical efficacy of FEIBA™ in spontaneous bleeds. Sjamsoedin et al. [3] studied the effect of FEIBA™ on joint and muscle bleeding in haemophilia A inhibitor patients. This randomised double-blind trial compared FEIBA™ with a non-activated PCC. Outcome comparison showed that FEIBA™ produced significant improvements in bleeding control and joint mobility. In 1983, Hilgartner and Knatterud described the outcomes of FEIBA™ use in 165 bleeding episodes in 49 inhibitor patients [4]. The majority of bleeds involved joints, but there were also 3 central nervous system bleeds and 4 surgical procedures. Ninety-three percent of bleeds were controlled, 36% with one infusion in 12 h and another 42% within 36 h. Hilgartner et al. later reported on the efficacy and safety of the second generation vapour-heated product, FEIBA-VH [5]. Seventy-nine percent of 106 bleeding episodes in inhibitor patients were controlled within 36 h, without significant toxicity. These results compared favourably with earlier studies and confirmed that the heat treating process did not alter efficacy. The largest observational trial on the use of FEIBA™ was a retrospective multi-centre French study [6]. Data was presented on 433 bleeding episodes, including surgical procedures, involving 60 patients. Efficacy was good or excellent in 81.3% and poor in 16.9% of treatment episodes. Tolerance was assessed as good in 98.8%, however an anamnestic response was noted in 31.5% of cases.

The first significant study reporting the use of Autoplex®T was by Kurczynski and Penner in 1974 [7]. Single doses of Autoplex®T were used to treat 60 bleeds in 8 severe haemophilia A inhibitor patients. Treatment was considered effective in most cases. A later study by Abildegard [8] used up to two doses of Autoplex®T within a 24-hour period to treat 25 bleeds in 9 severe haemophilia A inhibitor patients. Efficacy was reported at 88%. Multiple doses were effective in the treatment of 8 major bleeds occurring in 7 patients. Lusher et al. [9] conducted a controlled double-blind study to compare the effectiveness of Autoplex®T with Proplex, a prothrombin complex concentrate for the treatment of acute haemarthrosis. Efficacy at 6 h was just over 50% in all treatment groups and indicated that no additional benefit was derived from using the activated PCC. The largest study assessing the efficacy of Autoplex®T was reported by Kantrowitz et al. [10]. 454 infusions of Autoplex®T were used to treat 120 bleeding episodes in 60 severe haemophilia A patients with inhibitors. Autoplex®T was effective in the treatment of 87% of the bleeds.

Experience with aPCCs in Surgery

FEIBA™ and Autoplex®T have also been reported to be effective in providing cover for minor and major surgery and dental extractions in patients with inhibitors [6, 11]. The evidence base for use of FEIBA™ in surgery is restricted to only a few reports. Negrier et al [6] reported FEIBA™ was haemostatically effective in the treatment of 19 minor surgical procedures and effective in 4 major procedures in 3 patients. One patient had bilateral knee replacements and, subsequently, musculo-skeletal grafting. A second patient had a prostatectomy and a third patient had a full dental clearance. FEIBA™ was also reported to be effective as second-line treatment in 7 individuals who had undergone major surgical procedures complicated by development of anamnesis to either human or porcine factor VIII.

Published experience with the use of Autoplex®T in surgery on haemophilia A inhibitor patients is restricted to just one report [12]. Multiple doses of Autoplex®T effectively controlled haemostasis during a full dental clearance in 2 patients and a right forearm haematoma bleed in 1 patient.

Safety of aPCCs

Both FEIBA™ and Autoplex®T undergo viral inactivation procedures during manufacture [13]. The starting material for Autoplex®T undergoes an augmented Cohn alcohol fractionation and then the final product is dry heat treated for 6 days at 57 °C. FEIBA™ undergoes a two-stage vapour-heating treatment, initially for 10 h at 60 °C and then 1 h at 80 °C. Although FEIBA™ was associated with transmission of hepatitis B and C, there have been no reports of viral transmission since the introduction of viral inactivation procedures. Autoplex®T has not been associated with viral transmission.

Minor reactions have been reported in association with both FEIBA™ and Autoplex®T. These include headache, nausea, pruritus, skin rashes and diarrhoea. Such reactions were reported to have occurred in association with 8% of Autoplex®T infusions [10] and in 3.7% of FEIBA™ infusions [4].

Thrombotic complications including myocardial infarction and subclinical disseminated intravascular coagulation, although very rare, have been reported in association with FEIBA™, especially in patients undergoing surgery or in those who have received repeated high doses of the concentrate. A maximum daily dose of FEIBA™ of 200 U/kg has been recommended to minimise the risk of thrombogenicity. Moreover, the product should be avoided in patients with a history of vascular occlusive disease [14]. Although there has been no report of myocardial infarction or disseminated intravascular coagulation associated with the use of Autoplex®T as a single agent, the potential thrombogenetic risk of this product is recognised and concomitant treatment with antifibrinolytic agents should be avoided.

Anamnestic increases of inhibitor levels have been reported in up to 30% of patients with haemophilia A receiving FEIBA™, due to the presence of small amounts of FVIII in the product [15]. However, in over 50% of these patients who remain on regular FEIBA™ therapy the antibody level gradually falls. Autoplex®T has also been associated with the development of anamnestic responses in some patients. However, anamnestic responses to aPCCs are not associated with a reduction in the efficacy of these products.

Conclusion

Both FEIBA™ and Autoplex®T appear to be effective and safe in the management of bleeding episodes and surgery in haemophilia inhibitor patients. There is currently no laboratory test for monitoring the efficacy of aPCCs and dosage must be determined solely by clinical assessment. However, it is believed that the clinical effect of FEIBA™ may correlate with circulating thrombin generating potential and a fluorogenic substrate assay is being developed to enable monitoring of FEIBA™ dosage in vitro.

References

1 Turecek PL, Varadi K, Gritsch H, Schwarz HP: Activated prothrombin complex concentrates induce hemostasis by a balanced effect at multiple sites of the coagulation pathway. Haemophilia 1998;4:168 (abstract).

2 Lundblad RL, Bergstrom J, De Vreker R, Bray G, Gomperts E, Baker D, Kingdon HS, Mann KG, Hartshorn J, Jenny RJ: Measurement of active coagulation factors in Autoplex®-T with colorimetric active site-specific assay technology. Thromb Haemost 1998;80:811–815.

3 Sjamsoedin LJ, Heijnen L, Mauser-Bunschoten EP, van Geijlswijk JL, van Houwelingen H, van Asten P, Sixma JJ: The effect of activated prothrombin-complex concentrate (FEIBA) on joint and muscle bleeding in patients with haemophilia A and antibodies to factor VIII. A double-blind clinical trial. N Engl J Med 1981; 305:717–721.

4 Hilgartner MW, Knatterud GL: The use of factor eight inhibitor by-passing activity (FEIBA immuno) product for treatment of bleeding episodes in haemophiliacs with inhibitors. Blood 1983;61:36–40.

5 Hilgartner M, Aledort L, Andes A, Gill J: Efficacy and safety of vapor-heated anti-inhibitor coagulant complex in hemophilia patients. FEIBA study group. Transfusion 1990;30:626–630.

6 Negrier C, Goudemand J, Sultan Y, Bertrand M, Rothschild C, Lauroua P: Multicenter retrospective study on the utilization of FEIBA in France in patients with factor VIII and factor IX inhibitors. French FEIBA Study Group. Factor Eight Bypassing Activity. Thromb Haemost 1997;77:1113–1119.

7 Kurczynski EM, Penner JA: Activated prothrombin concentrate for patients with factor VIII inhibitors. N Engl J Med 1974;291:164–167.

8 Abildgaard CF, Penner JA, Watson-Williams EJ: Anti-inhibitor Coagulant Complex (Autoplex) for treatment of factor VIII inhibitors in hemophilia. Blood 1980;56:978–984.

9 Lusher JM, Blatt PM, Penner JA, Aledort LM, Levine PH, White GC, Warrier AI, Whitehurst DA: Autoplex versus proplex: A controlled, double-blind study of effectiveness in acute hemarthroses in hemophiliacs with inhibitors to factor VIII. Blood 1983;62:1135–1138.

10 Kantrowitz JL, Lee ML, McClure DA, Kingdon HS, Thomas WR: Early experience with the use of anti-inhibitor coagulant complex to treat bleeding in hemophiliacs with inhibitors to factor VIII. Clin Therapeut 1987;9:405–419.

11 Penner JA: Management of haemophilia in patients with high-titre inhibitors: Focus on the evolution of activated prothrombin complex concentrate AUTOPLEX T. Haemophilia 1999;5(suppl 3):1–9.

12 Hanna WT, Madigan RR, Miles MA, Lange RD: Activated factor IX complex in treatment of surgical cases of hemophilia A with inhibitors. Thromb Haemost 1981;46:638–641.

13 Horwith G, Revie DR: Efficacy of viral clearance methods used in the manufacture of activated prothrombin complex concentrates: Focus on AUTOPLEX T. Haemophilia 1999; 5(suppl 3):19–23.

14 Hay CRM, Baglin TP, Collins PW, Hill FGH, Keeling DM: The diagnosis and management of factor VIII and factor IX inhibitors: A guideline from the UK haemophilia center Doctors' organization (UKHCDO). Br J Haematol 2000;111.78–90.

15 Green D: Complications associated with the treatment of haemophiliacs with inhibitors. Haemophilia 1999;5(suppl 3):11–17.

Pathophysiology of Haemostasis and Thrombosis

Pathophysiol Haemost Thromb 2002;32(suppl 1):13–18

The Evidence behind Inhibitor Treatment with Recombinant Factor VIIa

Christopher A. Ludlam

Haemophilia and Thrombosis Centre, Royal Infirmary, Edinburgh, UK

Key Words

rFVIIa · Haemostatic response · Continuous infusion · Bolus dose

Abstract

Over the past 10 years considerable use has been made of recombinant factor VIIa (rFVIIa) for the treatment of patients with inhibitors to coagulation factors. During this time, its place in the management of acute bleeds and surgery has become better defined. Although pharmacokinetic studies report the half-life of rFVIIa as 2.7 h, there is considerable intersubject variability. Moreover, rFVIIa is cleared more rapidly in children than in adults. Assays for the measurement of rFVIIa plasma levels are not readily available in clinical diagnostic laboratories, although there is evidence that plasma FVII:C levels, measured by a one-stage prothombin-based assay, reflect the plasma concentration of rFVIIa:C. The level of FVII:C required to achieve haemostasis in different clinical circumstances remains uncertain. In order to overcome the logistic difficulties of repeated frequent bolus injections, and potentially to minimise usage, administration of rFVIIa by continuous infusion has been reported. However, there is some uncertainty as to whether continuous infusion of rFVIIa has similar therapeutic efficacy to an equivalent total dose administered by bolus injections. The extensive clinical experience with rFVIIa in haemophilic patients with inhibitors has been recorded in descriptive accounts of the Compassionate Use Programme and the Emergency Use Study. On the basis of the apparent clinical efficacy and safety reported in these studies, prospective randomised trials of different dose regimens have been undertaken for the treatment of acute bleeds and surgery. These have helped to define the minimum dose needed to achieve haemostasis. There remains considerable uncertainty about the minimal effective dose and appropriate duration of therapy in different clinical circumstances. There is therefore a need for the development of evidence-based guidelines for the use of rFVIIa in bolus and continuous infusion regimens in different settings, and for the therapeutic value of measuring plasma concentrations of rFVIIa, to facilitate the optimal use of this product. Furthermore, additional randomised clinical trials will help ensure that rFVIIa is used in the most clinically and cost effective way.

Introduction

Recombinant factor VIIa (rFVIIa) has been available for more than a decade. During this time, a wealth of experience has accumulated in the role of rFVIIa in managing haemophilia patients who have inhibitors to FVIII or IX. Such patients are resistant to conventional factor VIII concentrate therapy. Trials and case reports suggest that rFVIIa is effective in a variety of challenging clinical situations, including emergency treatment of acute bleeds, home treatment, and in acquired haemo-

KARGER

Fax + 41 61 306 12 34
E-Mail karger@karger.ch
www.karger.com

1424–8832/02/0327–0013$18.50/0

Accessible online at:
www.karger.com/journals/pht

Prof. Christopher Ludlam
Edinburgh Royal Infirmary
Department of Haematology, 1 Lauriston Place
Edinburgh, EH3 9YW (UK)
Tel. +44 131 536 2122, Fax +44 131 536 2145, E-Mail Christopher.Ludlam@ed.ac.uk

philia. It is coming under close scrutiny as a potential solution for those inhibitor patients who require surgery, an aspect of haemophilia care that is fraught with difficulties. Research is also focusing on dose regimens and on methods of administration of rFVIIa in an effort to determine the most effective and practical way of using the treatment.

This paper reviews the trial data for rFVIIa and highlights some of the questions that remain regarding the optimum use of this comcemtrate in the management of haemophilia patients with inhibitors.

Table 1. rVIIa Emergency Use Study 1996–1999

Patients	127
Bleeds	253
Dose	90 μg/kg 2-hourly
Efficacy	
Haemophilia A and B	93%
Acquired haemophilia	71%
Factor VII deficiency	89%

The Emergency Treatment Study, conducted 1996–1999, of the use of rFVIIa in 253 acute bleeds [5, 6].

Pharmacokinetics

Recombinant FVIIa has a short half life of 2.7 h in adults and only 1.3 h in children [1]. Clinical use of rFVIIa is further complicated by the fact that there is considerable variation in its pharmacokinetic behaviour between individual patients. This has led to suggestions that pharmacokinetic evaluation may be necessary for each patient.

Plasma levels of FVIIa can be measured with a conventional one-stage prothrombin-based, FVII:C assay. The level of FVII:C, hence the dose of rFVIIa, required to achieve haemostasis in different clinical settings is the subject of close investigation.

Early Clinical Studies

During the first 8 years that rFVIIa was available, patients received the agent under the Compassionate Use Programme [2–4]. Of 260 patients internationally who received rFVIIa in this programme between 1988 and 1996, 75% had haemophilia A or B, 14% had acquired haemophilia, and 11% had FVII deficiency. Over 1,000 bleeds were treated with rFVIIa given in bolus doses of 60–90 μg/kg. The efficacy was found to be 80–87% in serious bleeds and 91–94% in surgical bleeds.

The Compassionate Use Programme was followed by the 3-year Emergency Treatment Study, completing in 1999 [5, 6]. In this study, 253 acute bleeds in 127 patients were treated with rFVIIa, 90 μg/kg 2-hourly. The efficacy was 93% for haemophilia A or B patients with inhibitors and 71% for acquired haemophilia. In FVII-deficient patients the efficacy was 89% (table 1).

These promising results led to the first prospective randomised trials of various doses of rFVIIa in haemophilia patients with inhibitors.

Dose Finding Study

The first randomised, double-blind trial was an international dose-finding study of acute bleeds in severe haemophilia [7]. The multicentre trial involved 84 patients with 179 joint or muscle bleeds, of which 145 were evaluable. Patients received rFVIIa in a dose of 35 or 70 μg/kg in a parallel group design. Results showed that the two doses achieved similar rates of efficacy, which was graded as excellent or effective in 71% of bleeds. The mean number of doses given to the two groups was similar – 2.7 in the 35 μg/kg group and 3.1 in the 70 μg/kg group. These findings raised questions over optimum dosing for acute bleeds: either 35 μg/kg is adequate, or 70 μg/kg is inadequate.

Home Treatment Studies

Safety and efficacy of rFVIIa as home treatment have been confirmed by four major studies, involving a total of 102 patients and 864 bleeds [8–11]. Similar doses were used in each study, usually 90 μg/kg. Efficacy was approximately 90% in three of the studies and 79% in the fourth. The mean number of injections to obtain haemostasis was 2.2, although in the N American study an additional injection was given after the patients considered that they had stopped bleeding.

Delay to Treatment

In a review of intramuscular bleeds included in the Compassionate Use Study, the Dose-Finding Study and the US Home Treatment Study, it was found that the earlier the rFVIIa treatment is initiated, the better the clinical outcome [8–11] (table 2). During the Compassionate

Table 2. Comparison of time of treatment and response for peripheral intramuscular haemorrhages

	Dosage µg/kg	Time to treatment	Excellent or effective response, %	Mean number of doses of rFVIIa
Compassionate use	60–120	5 days	63.1	13.6
Dose finding	70	9 h	72	3.6
	35	9 h	53	3.5
US home treatment	90	1.2 h	92	2.3

Clinical response to rFVIIa treatment related to time from start of bleed [8–11].

Use Study, in which other treatments were tried first and rFVIIa was not given until day 5, an excellent or effective response was achieved in only 63% of intramuscular haemorrhages. In contrast, in the US Home Treatment Study in which the delay to rFVIIa treatment was only 1 h after the onset of the bleed, the response rate was 92%. There was a corresponding fall in the number of injections needed to achieve haemostasis – a mean of 13.6 injections in the Compassionate Use Study compared with only 2.3 in the US Home Treatment group.

Acquired Haemophilia

The benefit of starting rFVIIa treatment early after the onset of bleeding was shown again in a database analysis of 74 bleeding episodes in 38 patients with acquired haemophilia reported to Novo Nordisk [12]. Patients received rFVIIa as a first-line or salvage treatment for muscle haematoma, urinary/GI bleeds, haemarthroses, or surgery. A dose of 90 µg/kg was used, with a median of 28 doses given over approximately 4 days. For all 14 bleeding episodes where rFVIIa was received as first-line therapy, there was a good haemostatic response, compared with 75% of 60 bleeding episode where FVIIa was used as a salvage therapy.

Surgery

Smith and Hann were the first to describe the successful use of rFVIIa for central intravenous catheter insertion in children with haemophilia [13]. They used a 90 µg/kg dose of rFVIIa administered 2-hourly for 1 day and 4-hourly for a further 2 days, always with tranexamic acid. Their positive results have since been confirmed in a further study [14].

Other studies have attempted to establish the haemostatic dose of rFVIIa to prevent post-operative bleeding in haemophilia patients with inhibitors following surgery. One such study was a prospective double-blind trial comparing 35 µg/kg with 90 µg/kg of rFVIIa [14]. Patients were randomised to receive one of the two doses as a bolus injection, beginning pre-operatively, then 2-hourly for 2 days and 2–6 hourly for a further 3 days. Of the patients, 18 had minor surgery (all central venous catheter insertions) and 11 had major surgery, mostly orthopaedic. At 48 h after wound closure the results showed that for minor surgery, haemostasis was achieved in all 8 of those receiving the 90 µg/kg dose and in 9 of 10 patients receiving 35 µg/kg. Among the patients undergoing major surgery, all 6 patients receiving the higher dose and 3 of 5 receiving the lower dose achieved haemostasis.

For minor surgery, the median total dose of rFVIIa was slightly less for the 35 µg/kg dose group than for the 90 µg/kg dose (45 mg compared with 67 mg) (table 3). However, in patients undergoing major surgery, more rFVIIa was used in the low dose group than in those receiving the high dose (656 vs. 569 mg). Correspondingly, more injections of rFVIIa were needed in the major surgery patients allocated to low dose (median 135 vs. 81 in the high dose group), because of the patients who bled following the low dose. Treatment was given for a median of 15 days with the lower dose compared with 9.5 days for the higher dose. These findings reflect the fact that loss of haemostasis post-surgery can be extremely difficult to control. Therefore, using the lower dose of a coagulation therapy does not necessarily result in less of the drug being used over the course of the treatment period.

The authors concluded that while minor surgery was well controlled with bolus doses of 35 µg/kg of rFVIIa, major surgery needed 90 µg/kg.

Table 3. rVIIa 35 and 90 μg/kg boluses in surgery dosing

	Minor surgery		Major surgery	
	35 μg/kg (n = 10)	90 μg/kg (n = 7)	35 μg/kg (n = 5)	90 μg/kg (n = 6)
Median duration of				
Dosing, days	4.0	6.0	15.0	9.5
Range	3–6	3–6	2–26	8–17
Median number of				
Injections	29.5	38.0	135.0	81.0
Range	24–44	26–67.0	11–186	71–128
Median total dose of rFVIIA, mg	45.5	67.0	656	569
Range	14–171	31–122	31–839	107–698

A prospective double-blind trial comparing 35 μg/kg with 90 μg/kg of rFVIIa in patients undergoing surgery [14].

Table 4. rVIIa by CI at 50 μg/kg/h elective orthopaedic surgery

Bolus 90 μg/kg pre-operative
CI – 50 μg/kg/h
Duration – at investigators discretion
Bleeds – bolus 60 μg/kg
FVIIC – reached 30 IU/ml in 87%

Protocol for continuous infusion of rFVIIa at 50 μg/kg/h for orthopaedic surgery.

Administration

In view of the short half life of rFVIIa, continuous infusion has been investigated as a possible means of overcoming the logistical difficulties of administering frequent bolus injections and possibly to minimise the dose required.

An Italian study investigated the continuous infusion of rFVIIa in doses of 16–20 μg/kg/h in 35 patients with FVIII inhibitors [15]. Of the patients, 11 underwent major surgery, 14 had minor surgery and 10 had spontaneous bleeds. They received an initial bolus dose of approximately 100 μg/kg prior to continuous infusion at a dose determined by the attending physician. Median doses were 20 μg/kg/h for the patients undergoing major surgery, 17 μg/kg/h for those having minor surgery, and 16 mg/kg/h in the spontaneous bleeds group. Treatment was continued for 8 days following major surgery, 3 days after minor surgery, and 5 days for those with spontaneous bleeds.

Haemostasis was effective in 30 of the patients, partially effective in 2 and ineffective in 4 individuals. This study found that plasma FVII level did not appear to be related to the propensity to bleeding.

Continuous Infusion Dose

The relationship between efficacy and plasma levels of FVII was studied more closely by our group in a trial of 8 inhibitor patients undergoing elective surgery [16]. One of the aims of this study was to see whether a continuous infusion dose of 16.5 μg/kg/h would achieve FVII plasma levels of at least 10 IU/ml, believed at the time of the study to be the haemostatic level for FVIIa. Six patients had major surgery (joint replacement) and 2 had minor surgery (1 bladder biopsy, 1 central line insertion). They were given an initial bolus of 90 μg/kg pre-operatively followed immediately by the continuous infusion. If a patient bled, a bolus of 60 μg/kg rFVIIa was given.

The study showed that FVII:C of at least 10 IU/ml was achieved in approximately 90% of assays. However, the clinical outcome was disappointing. Haemostasis was satisfactory in only 3 of the 8 patients: 1 of the 2 patients undergoing minor surgery and 2 of the 6 patients having major surgery.

In the light of these results, we initiated a second study to see whether increasing the dose of continuous infusion of rFVIIa – thereby raising the plasma level of FVII – would lead to less post-operative bleeding. In this study the aim was to achieve a FVII level of 30 IU/ml. Computer modelling predicted that this would be achieved with an infusion of 50 μg/kg/h and this dose was therefore used in the study [17]. Of the 9 patients, 8 had major joint replacements and 1 an amputation. The patients received a 90 μg/kg bolus of rFVIIa pre-operatively prior to continuous infusion, the duration of which was at the investigator's discretion.

The FVII:C level of at least 30 IU/ml was achieved in almost 90% (table 4). Following surgery bleeding occurred in 6 patients but all except one settled with a single bolus of 60 μg/kg rFVIIa. All patients had a good clinical outcome from the surgery.

Thus the continuous infusion of 50 μg/kg/h results in a FVII:C of 30 IU/ml and this level of FVII is adequate to achieve haemostasis. In this study, patients received the infusions for a median of 20 days, but for non-trial clinical use it is likely that a shorter duration would suffice. Further investigation is needed to determine whether infusion rates could be reduced over the course of treatment, with corresponding decreasing FVII plasma levels but without losing haemostatic efficacy.

Adverse Events

Since registration in various countries until February 2001 it has been estimated that 171,790 doses of rVIIa had been sold. A total of 87 adverse events had been spontaneously reported in association with the use of marketed rVIIa. The list of adverse events includes decreased therapeutic response (16), cardiovascular events (17) which included myocardial infarction (7), cerebrovascular (6), venous thrombosis/thrombophlebitis (6) and disseminated intravascular coagulation (1). Seventeen patients who experienced a serious adverse event died and 8 were causally evaluated by the investigator to be possibly or probably related to the administration of rVIIa [18]. Further work is required to review these adverse events to define their causal relationship to rVIIa.

Comment

Evidence gained over the past 13 years demonstrates that rFVIIa has a role in the management of patients with haemophilia and inhibitors to coagulation factors. However, we do not yet know how best to use this agent, and several questions must be answered before it can be used optimally.

What Is the Minimum Effective Dose?

Perhaps the most pressing need is to identify the minimum dose of this expensive treatment that is needed to achieve haemostasis. The clinical trials have established that rFVIIa is effective for acute bleeds when given in boluses of 90 μg/kg 2–3-hourly. Major surgery can be accomplished successfully with boluses of 90 μg/kg every 2–4 h. Whether it is feasible to achieve a good response in orthopaedic surgery with smaller doses is yet to be determined. Minor surgery may be safely undertaken with lower doses. Given the importance of maximising the cost effectiveness of rFVIIa, further clinical trials to clarify optimum dose regimens warrant a high priority.

Optimal doses for continuous infusion also remain unclear. The Italian data suggest that rFVIIa is effective at 20 μg/kg/h even for major surgery. In contrast, the studies by our group indicate that, for major surgery, the dose needs to be 50 μg/kg/h.

Is Continuous Infusion Preferable to Bolus Therapy?

In determining whether the optimal approach is the 90 μg/kg bolus dose or the 20–50 μg/kg/h continuous infusion, it is important to consider the mechanism of action of rFVIIa. We do not currently know how rFVIIa achieves haemostasis, but there is a view that the key to successful treatment may be the burst of thrombin activity generated particularly by the bolus dose which promotes the formation of a strong fibrin clot at the bleeding site. Furthermore, it has recently been observed that high doses of thrombin are needed to activate TAFI, an inhibitor of thrombolysis [19].

The importance of platelets in the action of rFVIIa is supported by studies of platelet activation and platelet microparticles that are released following stimulation with thrombin. These studies led to the discovery that bolus doses of rFVIIa, particularly in combination with tranexamic acid, are associated with a rapid increase in platelet microparticles in haemophiliac patients [20]. Further research is needed to clarify the mechanism of action of rFVIIa and the role of tranexamic acid.

These questions point to an urgent need for further laboratory studies and clinical trials to optimise the use of rFVIIa.

References

1 Hedner U, Kristensen H, Berntorp E, Ljung R, Petrini P, Tengborn L: Pharmacokinetics of rFVIIa in children. Haemophilia 1998;4:244 (abstract).

2 Ingerslev J, Freidman D, Gasstineau D, Gilchrist G, Johnsson H, Lucas G, McPherson J, Preston E, Scheibel E, Shuman M: Major surgery in haemophilic patients with inhibitors using recombinant factor VIIa. Haemostasis 1996;26:118–123.

3 McPherson J, Teague L, Lloyd J, Jupe D, Rowell J, Ockelford P, Ekert H, Street A, Faase A, Hedner U: Experience with recombinant factor VIIa in Australia and New Zealand. Haemostasis 1996:26:109–117.

4 Scharrer I: Recombinant factor VIIa for patients with inhibitors to factor VIII or IX or factor VII deficiency. Haemophilia 1999:5:253–259.

5 Arkin S, Blei F, Fetten J, Foulke R, Gilchrist GS, Heisel MA, Key N, Kisker CT, Kitchen C, Shafer FE, Shah PC, Strickland D: Human coagulation factor FVIIa (recombinant) in the management of limb-threatening bleeds unresponsive to alternative therapies: Results from the NovoSeven emergency-use programme in patients with severe haemophilia or with acquired inhibitors Blood Coagul Fibrinolysis 2000;11:255–259.

6 Liebman HA, Chediak J, Fink KI, Galwez AG, Shah PC, Shann RL: Activated recombinant human coagulation factor VII therapy for abdominal bleeding in patients with inhibitory antibodies to factor VIII. Am J Hematol 2000; 63:109–113.

7 Lusher JM, Roberts HR, Davignon G, Joist JH, Smith H, Shapiro A, Laurian Y, Kasper CK, Mannucci PM: A randomised, double-blind comparison of two dosage levels of recombinant factor VIIa in the treatment of joint, muscle and mucotaneous haemorrhages in persons with haemophilia A and B, with and without inhibitors. Haemophilia 1998;4:790–798.

8 Ingerslev J, Thykjaer H, Kudsk Jensen O, Fredberg U: Home treatment with recombinant factor VII: results from one centre. Blood Coagul Fibrinolysis 1998;9(suppl 1):107–110.

9 Santagostino E, Gingeri A, Mannucci PM: Home treatment with recombinant activated factor VII in patients with factor VIII inhibitors: the advantages of early intervention. Br J Haematol 1999;104:22–26.

10 Laurian Y, Goudemand J, Négrier C et al: Use of recombinant activated factor VII as first line therapy for bleeding episodes in haemophiliacs with factor VIII or IX inhibitors. Blood Coagul Fibrinolysis 1998;9(suppl 1):155–156.

11 Key NS, Aledort LM, Beardsley D, Cooper HA, Davignon G, Ewenstein BM, Gilchrist GS, Gill JC, Glader B, Hoots WK, Kisker CT, Lusher JM, Rosenfield CG, Shapiro AD, Smith H, Taft E: Home treatment of mild to moderate bleeding episodes using recombinant factor VIIa (NovoSeven) in haemophiliacs with inhibitors. Thromb Haemost 1998;80:912–918.

12 Hay CRM, Negrier C, Ludlam CA: The treatment of bleeding in acquired haemophilia with recombinant factor VIIa: A multicentre study. Thromb Haemost 1997;78:1463–1467.

13 Smith OP, IM Hann: rVIIa therapy to secure haemostasis during central line insertion in children with high-responding FVIII inhibitors. Br J Haematol 1996;92:1002–1004.

14 Shapiro AD, Gilchrist GS, Hoots WK, Cooper A, Gastineau DA: Prospective, Randomised Trial of Two Doses of fFVIIa (NovoSeven) in Haemophilia Patients with InhibitorsUndergoing Surgery, Thromb Haemost 1998;80:773–778.

15 Santagostino E, Morfini M, Rocino A, Scaraggi FA, Gingeri A: Relationship between factor VII activity and clinical efficacy of recombinant factor VIIa given by continuous infusion to patients with factor VIII inhibitors. Thromb Haemost 2001;86:954–958.

16 Smith MP, Ludlam CA, Collins PW, Hay CR, Wilde JT, Gingeri A, Melsen T, Savidge GF: Elective surgery on factor VIII inhibitor patients using continuous infusion of recombinant activated factor VII: Plasma factor VII activity of 10 IU/ml Is associated with an increased incidence of bleeding. Thromb Haemost 2001;86:949–953.

17 Ludlam CA, Smith MP, Morfini M, Gringeri A, Santagostino E, Savidge GT: A prospective study of recombinant activated factor VII administered by continuous infusion to inhibitor patients undergoing elective major orthopaedic surgery: A pharmacokinetic and efficacy evaluation. In preparation.

18 Novo Nordisk data on file: Investigator's Brochure; Recombinant Coagulation Factor VIIa 10th Edition, 20 March 2001.

19 Bajzar l, Manuel R, Neshiem ME: Purification and characterization of TAFI, a thrombin-activatable fibrinolysis inhibitor. J Biol Chem 1995;270:14477–14484.

20 Proulle V, Hugel B, Gulliet B, Rafowicz A, d'Oiron R, Lambet T, Tchernia G, Freyssinet JM, Dreyfus M: Circulating microparticles as a marker of recombinant activated FVII (NovoSeven) efficacy in patients with FVIII or FIX inhibitors. J Thromb Haemost 2001(suppl): OC1771 (abstract).

Pathophysiology of Haemostasis and Thrombosis

Pathophysiol Haemost Thromb 2002;32(suppl 1):19–21

The 2000 United Kingdom Haemophilia Centre Doctors' Organisation (UKHCDO) Inhibitor Guidelines

C.R.M. Hay

Manchester Thrombosis and Haemostasis Centre, Manchester, UK

Key Words
Inhibitor · Guidelines · UKHCDO · Haemophilia

Abstract
The UKHCDO inhibitor guidelines address the diagnosis and management of patients with haemophilia A, haemophilia B and acquired haemophilia. Recommendations are based on best current practice as reflected in the published evidence base. Many current treatment strategies are based on uncontrolled observations highlighting the need for well designed controlled studies.

Introduction

The UKHCDO Guideline on the diagnosis and management of factor VIII and factor IX inhibitors derives from the contemporary evidence base, and represents a consensus agreed by directors of haemophilia comprehensive care centres throughout the United Kingdom [1]. The guideline provides a comprehensive and practical resource, addressing monitoring for inhibitors, laboratory diagnosis, approaches to immune tolerance induction, treatment of bleeding events and management of acquired haemophilia. Levels of evidence are those defined in AHCPR 1992 [2].

Inhibitor Monitoring and Diagnosis

The guideline recommends an APPT mixing/incubation test should be used for inhibitor screening. This is a sensitive but non-quantitative technique. The committee could not decide which of the different methods is optimal, in the absence of comparative data. Inhibitor quantification should use the Nijmegen modification of the Bethesda technique [3], as endorsed by the factor VIII and IX Scientific Subcommittee of the International Society of Thrombosis and Haemostasis [4]. Prophylactic concentrate administration should be optimized through periodic pharmacokinetic studies in individual patients. This approach incorporates some degree of surveillance for inhibitors. Often a reduced factor VIII recovery or a very low trough level during prophylaxis may be the first indicator of a low level inhibitor. The median time to development of an inhibitor is 9 to 12 exposure days [5]. For this reason inhibitor screening should be conducted initially every fifth exposure day or quarterly until the 20th exposure day, and thereafter every 6–12 months. This approach will allow early detection of low-level inhibitors, which might otherwise be missed.

Immune Tolerance Induction in Haemophilia A

Immune tolerance induction (ITI) should be considered for all newly diagnosed inhibitor patients. Such programmes should be conducted in centres with expertise

KARGER
Fax +41 61 306 12 34
E-Mail karger@karger.ch
www.karger.com

1424–8832/02/0327–0019$18.50/0

Accessible online at:
www.karger.com/journals/pht

Dr. Charles Richard Morris Hay
University Department of Haematology
Manchester Royal Infirmary, Oxford Road
Manchester, M13 9RY (UK)
Tel. +44 161 276 4812, Fax +44 161 276 4814, E-Mail haemophilia@man.ac.uk

and experience with this therapeutic strategy. Immune tolerance induction is a substantial financial undertaking. Interruptions to ITI are associated with increased failure rates. For this reason, realistic and appropriate funding for at least the first year should be secured in advance.

The impact of ITI on the patient and his family requires that informed consent be obtained before starting. After initial inhibitor diagnosis, the patient should not be exposed to further factor VIII until ITI begins. During this time bleeding episodes should be treated with recombinant factor VIIa (rFVIIa) until the inhibitor titre has declined to less than 10 BU/ml. Studies show that the prognosis for success is improved if the inhibitor titre is lower than 10 BU/ml when ITI is commenced [6, 7]. Because tolerance induction is primarily a therapeutic strategy applied to children, it is recommended that recombinant factor VIII or IX be used, as this is consistent with the UKHCDO national guidelines and with Department of Health policy in the United Kingdom. Regardless of the inhibitor titre at the outset, most patients demonstrate an anamnestic response in the early phase of ITI, and become completely refractory to factor VIII for a period. Inhibitor bypassing therapy should be available to treat breakthrough bleeds during this time.

The optimal dose for good risk patients is unresolved and is the subject of a forthcoming international study. Poor risk patients, those with very high-level inhibitors and whose inhibitor titre is greater than 10 BU/ml when they commence ITI, are probably best tolerised using a high dose regime (greater than 100 IU/kg per day). A good risk patient is defined as under the age of five, with a starting inhibitor titre less than 10 BU/ml and an historical peak titre of less than 100 to 200 BU/ml [6, 7]. One of the commonest reasons to interrupt therapy is the onset of central line infection, associated with non-specific stimulation of the immune system and a rise in the inhibitor titre. Infections also lead to interruption of therapy, which may adversely influence outcome and should be avoided wherever possible [7].

Treatment of Bleeding

The choice of haemostatic product is based on the clinical bleeding severity, any historic anamnestic response, the clinical response to the various products the patient has previously been exposed to and the current inhibitor titre. Low responders have inhibitor levels of less than 5 BU/ml and do not develop an anamnestic response on further exposure to factor VIII. High responders have historical inhibitor titres greater than 5 BU/ml, and demonstrate an anamnestic rise in their inhibitor titre when re-exposed to factor VIII.

In low responders the therapeutic options would usually be human or porcine factor VIII, rFVIIa or FEIBA. Many low responders can be maintained successfully on human factor VIII at increased dose. In the case of a high level high responding patient, human or porcine factor VIII should be reserved for life or limb-threatening bleeding events. For all other bleeding events in this patient category, rFVIIa or FEIBA are indicated. In the UK and Ireland rFVIIa is recommended as the treatment of first choice for children unresponsive to factor VIII, because of its recombinant status and favourable side-effect profile. All major bleeding events should be managed with the product most likely to produce a rapid response.

Surgery

Surgery for inhibitor patients is a high-risk procedure, and is best undertaken in an experienced centre. Human or porcine factor VIII may be used if satisfactory factor VIII levels can be achieved. In congenital as opposed to acquired haemophilia, the clinical response to porcine factor VIII correlates with the factor VIII recovery [8]. There is no conclusive evidence that rFVIIa is significantly thrombogenic. Published reports of rFVIIa use for elective surgery are accumulating. It is therefore recommended rFVIIa is first-line treatment for patients in whom a satisfactory factor VIII level cannot be achieved. There is comparatively little data on the use of FEIBA for surgery.

Factor IX Inhibitors

When considering the management of factor IX inhibitors, the central variable is whether or not they suffer from anaphylaxis. This complicates management considerably. Those with a low inhibitor titre without anaphylaxis can be successfully managed with factor IX, FEIBA or rFVIIa. High responder patients are generally refractory to factor IX, and require rFVIIa or FEIBA. National treatment policy dictates that rFVIIa is the treatment of choice for children in the UK and Ireland unresponsive to or reacting to factor IX. For minor bleeding, preference may be given to products unlikely to cause anamnesis. Recombinant FVIIa is the treatment of choice for patients who have demonstrated anaphylaxis, as these reactions can be life-threatening.

ITI for factor IX inhibitor patients is more difficult and less successful than is the case for haemophilia A. In those without anaphylaxis, high purity or recombinant factor IX is recommended to avoid the thrombotic adverse events associated with intermediate purity products. At least the first few doses should be administered in hospital in case anaphylaxis occurs. Allergic reactions arise after a median of 11 exposure days in the treatment history. Pre-medication is often only partly effective in suppressing the reactions. Patients with anaphylaxis on ITI programmes may develop nephrotic syndrome, and this condition should be monitored for [9]. This may not resolve completely when factor IX therapy is discontinued.

Acquired Haemophilia

Acquired haemophilia commonly presents from medical or surgical specialties. It is recommended experienced centres should manage these patients, particularly when bleeding complications occur. Mortality from haemorrhage has been reported in up to 22% of cases [10]. For this reason, the guideline emphasises that immunosuppressive therapy should start immediately. First line treatment should be a combination of prednisolone and cyclophosphamide. In cases of inadequate response second line treatment options include high dose immunoglobulin, cyclosporine or multiple agent chemotherapy. Immunoabsorption may be a very useful adjunct in these patients, given at the same time as the initial immunosuppression.

Human factor VIII is usually ineffective for the treatment of bleeding in acquired haemophilia. Similarly DDAVP is usually ineffective unless the inhibitor level is so low that the patient has a measurable residual factor VIII. Significant bleeding should be treated aggressively. The treatment of choice is either rFVIIa or, if available, porcine factor VIII because of the relatively low cross-reactivity. Cross-reactivity as indicated by the Bethesda assay is at best semi-quantitative in this clinical context. More minor bleeding can be treated with rFVIIa, porcine factor VIII or FEIBA.

Conclusion

Most of the evidence for recommendations in this area is grade III or IV. All newly diagnosed inhibitors should be tolerised if possible. The optimal method for immune tolerance induction is disputed and trials are needed. The relative efficacy of different haemostatic treatment options are not well established and comparative studies would be very useful. Finally, effort should be directed to optimizing the contractual mechanism for funding immune tolerance induction programmes. Such consideration will inevitably involve assessment of cost-effectiveness of such therapy for different risk groups, together with analysis of risk-sharing strategies.

Acknowledgement

The inhibitor guidelines were drafted by UKHCDO inhibitor working party: CRM Hay, TP Baglin, PW Collins, FGH Hill and DM Keeling and subsequently ratified by the UKHCDO Executive Committee.

References

1 Hay CRM, Baglin TP, Collins PW, Hill FGH, Keeling DM: The diagnosis and management of factor VIII and factor IX inhibitors: A guideline from the UK haemophilia center Doctors' organization (UKHCDO). Br J Haematol 2000;111:78–90.

2 AHCPR (1992) Acute pain management: Operative or medical procedures and trauma. Agency of healthcare policy and research publications. United States Department of Health and Human Services, Washington.

3 Verbruggen B, Novakova I, Wessels H, Boezman J, van den Berg M, Mauser-Bunschoten E: The Nijmegan modification of the Bethesda assay for factor VIII:C inhibitors: Improved specificity and reliability. Thromb Haemost 1995;73:247–250.

4 Giles A, Verbruggen B, Rivard G, Teitel J, Walker I: A detailed comparison of the performance of the standard versus the Nijmegen modification of the Bethesda assay in detecting factor VIII:C inhibitors in the haemophilia A population of Canada. Thromb Haemost 1998; 79:872–876.

5 Ehrenforth S, Kreuz W, Scharrer I, Linde R, Funk M, Gungor T, Krackhardt B, Kornhuber B: Incidence of development of factor VIII and factor IX inhibitors in haemophiliacs. Lancet 1992;339:594–598.

6 DiMichele DM, Kroner BL & the ISTH factor VIII/IX sub-committee: Analysis of the North American immune tolerance registry (NAITR)(1993–97); Current practice implications. Vox Sang 1999;77:31–32.

7 Lenk H & the Study Group of the German Haemophilia Centres: The German National Immune Tolerance Registry, 1997 update. Vox Sang 1999;77:28–30.

8 Morrison AE, Ludlam CA, Kessler C: Use of porcine factor VIII in the treatment of patients with acquired haemophilia. Blood 1993;81: 1513–1520.

9 Wenstein BM, Takemoto C, Warrier I, Lusher J, Saidi P, Eisle J, Ettinger LJ, DiMichele DM: Nephrotic syndrome as a complication of immune tolerance in hemophilia B. Blood 1997; 89:1115–1116.

10 Hay CRM, Negrier C, Ludlam CA: The treatment of bleeding in acquired haemophilia with recombinant factor VIIa. Thromb Haemost 1997;78:1463–1467.

Pathophysiology of Haemostasis and Thrombosis

Pathophysiol Haemost Thromb 2002;32(suppl 1):22–25

Recombinant Factor VIIa in the Management of Surgery and Acute Bleeding Episodes in Children with Haemophilia and High-Responding Inhibitors

Owen P. Smith

National Centre for Hereditary Coagulation Disorders, The National Children's Hospital, Dublin, and St. James's Hospital, Dublin, Ireland

Key Words
Children · Inhibitors · Surgery · Bleeding episodes

Abstract
The development of inhibitors to therapeutic factor concentrates in children with haemophilia A or B is a troublesome complication of factor replacement therapy. Immune tolerance protocols have been developed to eliminate the inhibitors, and these are successful in approximately 80% of children. However, acute bleeding episodes require treatment with a factor (F)VIII or FIX bypassing agent to prevent an anamnestic rise in the inhibitor level before starting immune tolerance. In addition, central venous access is necessary to help parents administer frequent, high dose factor concentrate. In view of the benefits of rFVIIa seen in adults, a study has been carried out on the use of this agent as haemostatic cover in children with severe FVIII or FIX deficiency with high responding inhibitors. Information was obtained retrospectively from the National Children's Hospital, Dublin and Great Ormond Street Hospital, London. Twelve children aged 1–16 years were treated successfully with rFVIIa to prevent surgical bleeding in 20 surgical procedures. Minor post-operative haematomata developed in 2 of 20 cases after regular rFVIIa therapy had been discontinued. In both cases, resolution of bleeding occurred after a short course of rFVIIa. Three children experienced a total of six life- or limb-threatening bleeds. All bleeding episodes resolved with regular rFVIIa treatment, although topical fibrin glue was needed in one child with a frenulum tear. The rFVIIa therapy was well tolerated and there was no evidence of any treatment-related complications. In conclusion, rFVIIa is the treatment of choice for the management of surgery and acute life- or limb-threatening bleeding in children with haemophilia and high responding inhibitors.

Introduction

Inhibitor formation is a serious complication of haemophilia therapy as it impairs the efficacy of factor replacement treatment. Patients with high titre inhibitors fail to respond to factor concentrates even if high doses of the treatment are used. Patients most at risk of inhibitor development are those with previously untreated haemophilia, usually children with severe haemophilia A. The incidence of inhibitors approaches 33% in patients with FVIII deficiency and 3% of those with FIX deficiency [1].

KARGER

Fax + 41 61 306 12 34
E-Mail karger@karger.ch
www.karger.com

1424–8832/02/0327–0022$18.50/0

Accessible online at:
www.karger.com/journals/pht

Dr. Owen Smith
Medical Director/Consultant Haematologist
National Centre for Hereditary Coagulation Disorders
St James's Hospital, Dublin 8 (Ireland)
Tel. +353 1453 7941, Fax +353 1410 3475, E-Mail osmith@stjames.ie

Several publications have shown that immune tolerance therapy (ITT) can ablate the inhibitors in 80% of children who develop them [2–5]. Immune tolerance is more likely to succeed if the patient has an inhibitor titre less than 10 Bethesda Units (BU). However, acute bleeding episodes continue to require adequate haemostatic cover with a FVIII- or FIX-bypassing agent to prevent an anamnestic rise in the inhibitor level before starting ITT. In addition, young children require the insertion of a central venous access catheter, again with haemostatic cover, to help parents administer frequent high dose factor concentrate and acute treatment. The provision of this haemostatic cover can be achieved with rFVIIa. To date, the use of rFVIIa has been predominantly in adults with severe FVIII-deficiency and inhibitors who are undergoing surgery [6]. The agent has also become established as the treatment of choice for acute life-threatening bleeding episodes in adult haemophilia patients with inhibitors.

In the light of the experience with rFVIIa in adults, there has been much interest over the past few years in the use of this agent in paediatric patients who have severe FVIII-or FIX-deficiency with inhibitors. A study has therefore been carried out to investigate the use of rFVIIa in the management of surgery and acute bleeding episodes in children with haemophilia and high responding inhibitors [7].

Table 1. Study design for the two-centre investigation of the use of rFVIIa in the management of surgery and acute bleeds in children with haemophilia and inhibitors

- rFVIIa usage in children with sFVIII/IX and inhibitors Dec 1995 to Dec 2000.
- Retrospective via chart review
- rFVIIa dosage used for acute bleeds:
  - 90 μg/kg 2–4 h until bleeding stopped (TxA 15 mg/kg, topicalfibrin glue in 1 patient)
- rFVIIa dosage for surgical cover:
  - 90 μg/kg, 2 h × 24 h, 4 h × 24 h (NCH)
  - 90 μg/kg, 2 h × 24 h, 3 h × 24 h, 4 h × 24 h (GOS) (TxA 15 mg/kg i.v. or p.o. × 1 week)
- Efficacy – clinical assessment/shortening of PT

Table 2. Patient characteristics of participants in the London/Dublin study

Median age, years	2.5
Range	1–16
FVIII	12
FIX	1
Max. historical BU	
Median	120
Range	2–712
BU at time of rFVIIa	
Median	12
Range	<1–100

Study Design

The study was a retrospective chart review by the National Children's Hospital in Dublin and the Great Ormond Street Hospital for Children in London. The review included children with haemophilia and inhibitors who received rFVIIa between December 1995 and December 2000. During this time, 12 children received rFVIIa for the prevention of bleeding during a total of 20 surgical procedures (table 1). Additionally, rFVIIa treatment was given to 3 children among whom there were 6 acute life- or limb-threatening bleeding episodes.

Regimen

For the surgical cover, the dose of rFVIIa used in the Dublin centre was 90 μg/kg every 2 h during the first 24 h and then every 4 h during the following 24 h. At Great Ormond Street, the dose used for surgical cover was 90 μg/kg 2-hourly for the first day, 3-hourly for the second day and 4-hourly for the third day. The acute bleeding episodes were treated with a dose of rFVIIa of 90 μg/kg every 2–4 h until the bleeding stopped. All these patients also received tranexamic acid in a dose of 15 mg/kg either intravenously or orally for 1 week.

Efficacy was measured by clinical assessment of haemostasis. Shortening of the prothrombin time was also measured.

Patient Characteristics

The patients in this study had a median age of 2.5 years, ranging from 1 to 16 years (table 2). Of the patients, 12 were FVIII-deficient and one was FIX-deficient. The patients' records showed that their median maximum historical inhibitor titre was 120 BU with a range of 2–712 BU. At the time of rFVIIa treatment, the median inhibitor level was 12 BU with a range of 1–100 BU.

Surgery

The operations included 19 procedures for insertion or removal of a central venous access device (CVAD) and

Table 3. Surgical procedures

Number of patients	12
Total number of procedures	20
CVAD insertion or removal	19
Multiple dental extractions	1
Duration of cover, h	
Median	48
Range	12–72
Total dose rFVIIa, mg	
Median	43.2
Range	19.2–124.8

Table 4. Acute life-threatening bleeding episodes

Number of patients	3
Total number of bleeds	6
Mouth bleed	3
Port bleed	2
Forearm bleed/neuro $ms	1
Duration of cover, h	
Median	20
Range	4–96
Total dose rFVIIa, mg	
Median	43.2
Range	2.4–46.8

one multiple dental extraction (table 3). The median duration of surgical cover with rFVIIa was 48 h, ranging from 12–72 h. The median total dose of rFVIIa for surgery was 43 mg with a range of 19–125 mg.

All the surgical patients were treated successfully with rFVIIa. Two of the patients had minor bleeding 3 days after insertion of their CVAD, at which time both had discontinued their rFVIIa treatment. Re-treatment with 2–3 doses of rFVIIa resolved the bleeding.

Acute Bleeding

The 6 acute bleeds that occurred in 3 patients included mouth bleeds in 3 patients and port bleeds in 2 patients following insertion of a needle. One child had a forearm bleed with neurological symptoms. Three of the 6 bleeding episodes were associated with significant anaemia, haemoglobin levels dropping below 8 g/dl. Transfusion of red blood cells was required in 2 of the bleeding episodes.

Patients in the acute bleed group received rFVIIa treatment over a median of 20 h, ranging from 4–96 h (table 4). The median total dose of rFVIIa in these patients was 43 mg, ranging from 2–47 mg. All the bleeding episodes resolved with rFVIIa treatment, except one case involving a frenulum tear, which was brought under control by application of topical fibrin glue.

Prothrombin Time

Prothrombin time (PT) was measured in all 20 surgical procedures and in 1 of the patients with acute bleeds. In all 21 occasions, the PT shortened to the lower limit of normal following rFVIIa treatment. It was assumed this confirmed that a haemostatic level of FVII:C had been reached.

Side Effects

Treatment with rFVIIa was well tolerated. No treatment-related complications were seen in any of these surgical or acute bleed cases. There was no evidence of systemic activation of coagulation as indicated by activation markers including a D-Dimer.

Conclusion

We concluded from this series that rFVIIa was shown to be extremely effective and reliable in the management of acute bleeding episodes and in the prevention of surgical bleeding in children with FVIII- or FIX-deficiency with inhibitors.

Further research is required to determine the optimum therapeutic dose of rFVIIa in the paediatric setting. As the half-life of rFVIIa in children is only half that in adults, it could be that a lower bolus dose of rFVIIa would be effective. In assessing the best dose regimen, it may be necessary to examine more closely the kinetics of FVII:C in haemophiliac children with inhibitors during rFVIIa treatment. In this study, we noted that increasing the dosing intervals to 4-hourly was associated with a drop in the FVII:C levels which no longer exceeded the threshold believed to be necessary for haemostasis.

References

1 Hay CR, Baglin TP, Collins PW, Hill FG, Keeling DM: The diagnosis and management of factor VIII and factor IX inhibitors: A guideline from the UK Haemophilia Doctors' Organization (UKHCDO). Br J Haematol 2000;111:78–90.

2 Kreuz W, Ehrenforth S, Funk M, Auerswald D, Mentzer J, Joseph-Steiner J, Beeg T, Klarmann D, Scharrer I, Kornhuber B: Immune tolerance therapy in paediatric haemopiliacs with factor VIII inhibitors: 14 years follow-up. Haemophilia 1995;1:24–32.

3 Mauser-Bunschoten EP, Nieuwenhuis HK, Roosendaal G, van den Berg HM: Low-dose immune tolerance induction in hemophilia A patients with inhibitors blood 1995;86:983–988.

4 Di Michele DM: Immune Tolerance: A synopsis of the international experience. Haemophilia 1998;4:568–573.

5 Brackmann HH, Effenberger E, Hess L, Schwaab R, Oldenburg J: NovoSeven® in immune tolerance therapy. Blood Coagul Fibrin 2000;11(suppl 1):39–44.

6 Lusher J, Ingersley J, Roberts H, Hedner U: Clinical experience with recombinant factor VIIa. Blood Coagul Fibrin 1998;9:119–128.

7 O'Connell N, McMahon C, Smith J, Khair K, Hann I, Liesher R, Smith OP: Recombinant factor VIIa in the management of surgery and acute bleeding episodes in children with haemophilia and high responding inhibitors. Br J Haematol 2001;116:632–635.

Pathophysiology of Haemostasis and Thrombosis

Pathophysiol Haemost Thromb 2002;32(suppl 1):26–28

High Cost Patients and the Consortium Approach

Susan Schonfield[a] Keith Reid[b]

[a]Merton, Sutton & Wandsworth Health Authority, Mitcham, and [b]NHS Executive, London Regional Office, UK

Key Words

High cost patients · Commissioning consortium · Audit · Haemophilia A · Treatment

Abstract

The Pan-Thames Haemophilia Consortium was established to provide coherent regional planning of haemophilia services. The Expert Advisory Group is a clinical reference point for the consortium and was established to consider specifically elective high cost treatment programmes. An audit of the first year of consortium activity demonstrated that patients receiving high cost therapy represented 1.6% of the patient population and received 16% of the entire treatment budget. The Pan-Thames Consortium provides focused commissioning expertise and a model for national commissioning of haemophilia services.

Introduction

Specialized services are defined as high-cost, low volume services, needing at least one million population for an adequate burden of disease. In 1997 the new Labour government of the United Kingdom acknowledged that commissioning of specialized services had failed to work in the internal market environment of the National Health Service [1]. The White Paper quoted a report by the Audit Commission, which concluded that delivery of specialized services had been fragmented during the internal market, and now required stable and coherent regional planning with particular regard to organization and investment [2]. HSC (health service circular) 1998/198 [3] gave effect to this policy and recommended the formation of regional specialist commissioning groups (RSCGs) who would oversee the arrangements for planning, procuring and managing these services.

The Pan-Thames Haemophilia Consortium

This is one of the first consortia set up by the London RSCG and was formed in April 2000. The Pan-Thames Haemophilia Consortium commissions services from haemophilia Comprehensive Care Centres (CCCs) serving London and the surrounding regions of Kent, Surrey, Sussex, Hertfordshire and Essex. This area includes 24 health authorities, and covers a population of 13 million inhabitants. The Consortium aims to provide a coordinated and strategic approach to the commissioning of haemophilia services through planning of a service model, procurement of an agreed service specification and performance monitoring. It is led by Croydon Health Authority and comprises four sub-groups: strategy, finance, information and clinical. It is the work of the clinical subgroup that will be described in this paper.

KARGER

Fax + 41 61 306 12 34
E-Mail karger@karger.ch
www.karger.com

1424–8832/02/0327–0026$18.50/0

Accessible online at:
www.karger.com/journals/pht

Dr. Susan Schonfield
Merton, Sutton & Wandsworth Health Authority, The Wilson, Cranmer Road 6
Mitcham, Surrey CR4 4TP (UK)
Tel. +44 20 8687 4801, Fax +44 20 8687 4536
E-Mail susan.schonfield@mswha.sthames.nhs.uk

The Clinical Expert Advisory Group (EAG)

This group was formed to provide expert advice on the very high cost treatment programmes required by haemophilia patients who have acquired neutralising allo-antibodies (inhibitors) to coagulation factors. These treatments may relate to elective procedures such as operations or to immune tolerance induction. High cost was defined as those treatments with a concentrate purchase value of at least £100,000 in a three-month period.

Membership of the EAG comprises clinicians from four London CCCs, two public health specialists (one a former haematology consultant), two patient representatives, one haemophilia specialist nurse (from outside the Thames region) and one commissioning manager.

Initial tasks for the EAG involved establishing terms of reference and developing referral guidelines, including a patient information leaflet and consent form. The group only considers proposals for elective treatment and all patient referrals are presented anonymously. The clinical advice agreed on is communicated to the patient's health authority, with the letter copied to the clinician and, if requested, to the patient. The health authority then decides whether it wishes to accept the group's advice.

Clinical Audit

An audit of high cost patients treated in the first year of the Consortium (2000–2001) has recently been completed [4]. The audit objective was to identify the features of treatment programmes leading to high costs and to inform decisions on the purchase of haemophilia services. The study population included all patients with haemostatic disorders who received coagulation factor concentrate under the guidance of CCCs within the Haemophilia Consortium. The patients were categorised according to the cost of their coagulation factor concentrate use during the year. Specific clinical indications for individual high cost patients were then clarified through communication with the respective haemophilia treatment centres.

During the audit period, approximately 900 patients received coagulation concentrate treatment with a total cost of £38 million. For 96 of the 900 patients, treatment costs were in excess of £100,000 over the 12-month period. Fourteen patients (1.6%) satisfied the criteria of a high-cost patient, each receiving concentrate valued in excess of £100,000 over a 3-month period. The cost of their treatment accounted for 16% (£6,167,000) of the total concentrate budget. Of the 13 evaluable high-cost patients, 10 had severe haemophilia A (factor VIII less than 1 IU/dl), 1 had moderate haemophilia A (factor VIII 2–5 IU/dl) and 2 had mild haemophilia A (factor VIII greater than 5 IU/dl). Two patients were sero-positive for the HIV virus, one of which was co-infected with the hepatitis C virus. Four patients were sero-negative for the HIV virus but sero-positive for the hepatitis C virus. Nine of the 13 patients had inhibitory antibodies to factor VIII.

The treatment regimes of these 13 high-cost patients were listed as follows: 4 patients without factor VIII inhibitors were receiving regularly scheduled factor VIII concentrate in a prophylactic manner; 3 inhibitor patients were undergoing immune tolerance induction programmes with the aim of eradicating their inhibitory antibody; 4 patients were receiving inhibitor bypassing agents as required in response to bleeding episodes; and 2 patients received inhibitor bypassing agents for specific clinical problems, in one patient for the management of an infected joint prosthesis and in the other treatment for fulminant hepatic failure following an episode of variceal bleeding.

Two of the 4 patients receiving prophylactic factor VIII concentrate were teenagers of higher than average body weight, who had not yet undergone bone fusion of epiphyseal growth plates. They were receiving appropriate doses of recombinant factor VIII concentrate. One adult was receiving prophylaxis with plasma derived factor VIII concentrate, the clinical indications for which were not clear. Two of the 3 patients on immune tolerance induction programmes were children. One had successfully achieved full immune tolerance following initial central line insertion under recombinant factor VIIa cover. The other had achieved only partial success at immune tolerance induction following both high and intermediate dose regimes and continued on three times per week factor VIII concentrate therapy as a low dose immune tolerance induction regime, with recombinant factor VIIa as required for acute bleeding episodes. The third patient was an adult whose immune tolerance programme had failed and been discontinued, with reversion to a plasma derived inhibitor bypassing agent as required to treat bleeding episodes.

Discussion

The treatment categories for high cost patients included both the management of bleeding episodes and acute surgery for patients with specific coagulation factor inhibitors, immune tolerance induction programmes for patients with inhibitors, and appropriate prophylactic factor VIII replacement programmes for young adults of large body weight. Six of the 13 high cost treatment episodes were considered emergencies and the remaining seven were elective treatments. Two of these cases had been referred to the EAG for consideration. It should be noted that the EAG had started to receive referrals towards the end of the financial year covered by the retrospective audit.

The clinical advisory role of the EAG is still developing and several questions arise in terms of risk-sharing. These include under what circumstances would a health authority refuse to accept the clinical advice of the EAG, and whether all patients identified through financial returns to the consortium who meet the high cost criteria should be referred to the EAG. The audit shows that not all elective high cost cases were automatically referred to the group for consideration. A more consistent practice in referral of high cost treatment programmes for EAG consideration will be facilitated by improved data collection and outcome monitoring for this high cost but low volume caseload.

Declaration of Interests

Dr. Susan Schonfield's attendance at the Evidence Based Haemostasis seminar was funded by Croydon Health Authority and her speaker's honorarium will be paid to Croydon Health Authority. Dr. Keith Reid's attendance was funded by the London Region Public Health Training Programme.

References

1 'The New NHS – Modern, Dependable'. Department of Health, London, 1997, § 7.23.
2 'Higher Purchase: Commissioning Specialist Services in the NHS'. Audit Commission, London 1997.
3 HSC (health service circular) 1998/198. Department of Health, London, 1998.
4 Reid K, Schonfield S: Review of haemophilia patients deemed 'high-cost' conducted for the Pan Thames Haemophilia Consortium. Seville WFH, May 2002, poster in preparation.

Pathophysiology of Haemostasis and Thrombosis

Pathophysiol Haemost Thromb 2002;32(suppl 1):29–32

Economic Impact of Treating Inhibitor Patients

Loretto Lacey

Lacey Solutions Ltd, Dublin, Ireland

Key Words
Cost · Inhibitors · rFVIIa · QALY

Abstract
A literature review of the economics of managing haemophilia patients with inhibitors was conducted. It showed that haemophilia with inhibitors places a burden on the healthcare system and on the patient. Use of rFVIIa compared to 'usual therapy' is associated with improvements on a number of outcomes, including speed of bleed resolution, duration of pain, and quality of life. The extra costs of rFVIIa can be justified by the additional benefits achieved: For example, the extra costs required to achieve a gain of one quality adjusted life year (QALY) in children with inhibitors has been shown to be comparable with that for other reimbursed healthcare strategies. Future research could focus on expanding our understanding of the impact of accelerated bleed resolution on long-term sequelae, including need for surgery and quality of life.

Introduction

The management of bleeding episodes and surgery in haemophilia patients who develop inhibitors is especially difficult and expensive. As healthcare funding is a limited resource, management of these patients has to compete with other illnesses that also depend on expensive treatments and specialized staff. But it would be wrong to focus only on costs as new haemostatic agents offer many benefits to these patients. Consideration of the economics (i.e. costs and benefits) of treatment options in patients with inhibitors is, therefore, warranted. This paper reviews current publications on the economics of managing bleeding and surgery in haemophilia patients with inhibitors. A summary of the types and purposes of economic evaluations is presented along with some conclusions that can be drawn about the economics of treating inhibitor patients.

Overview of the Types and Purposes of Economic Analysis

With the exception of cost of illness and budget impact evaluations, economic evaluations invariably attempt to ascertain whether any additional costs associated with particular strategies are justified by additional benefits. Tables 1summarises the different forms of economic evaluations and how they inform the healthcare decision making process. The specific form of analysis used will be dictated by the question set.

Cost of illness (COI) analysis determines the cost of managing a particular cohort or defined population, identifying cost distribution and main cost drivers. Budget Impact Analysis (BIA) determines the financial impact of purchasing a new treatment for an indication or extending

KARGER
Fax + 41 61 306 12 34
E-Mail karger@karger.ch
www.karger.com

1424–8832/02/0327–0029$18.50/0

Accessible online at:
www.karger.com/journals/pht

Dr. Loretto Lacey
The Beaches, South Strand
Skerries, Co. Dublin (Ireland)
Tel./Fax +353 1 849 2420, E-Mail loretto@laceysolutions.com

Table 1. Economic evaluations inform decisions

Economic evaluation	Costs	Consequences	Decision rule
Cost of illness/budget impact	yes	no	affordability
Cost-consequences	yes	yes list all benefits	subjective
Cost-minimization	yes	yes pre-defined effectiveness outcome	the least costly way of achieving effect is recommended
Cost-effectiveness	yes	yes e.g. controlled bleed on 1st line	if ratio of additional cost to additional benefits less than £x, recommend use
Cost-utility	yes	yes, QALY gained	if additional cost per QALY gained less than £x, recommend use

the use of a currently subsidized drug to other indications/populations. Whilst COI and BIA only consider costs, they complement full economic evaluations because they address one major concern of healthcare decision-makers, remaining within the annual budget [1]! Full economic evaluations examine the costs and benefits of treatments. The simplest form, cost-consequences analysis lists all the costs and consequences associated with alternative treatment strategies [2]. Cost-minimisation analysis compares the cost of alternative treatment regimens producing the same outcome. Total costs, including the price of the drugs and costs associated with administration and management of adverse events, are determined. Cost-effectiveness analysis compares at least two treatment options and benefits are described in terms of illness specific outcomes [e.g. bleeds avoided, bleeds controlled with 1st line treatment). 'Value for money' is informed by the ratio of additional costs relative to additional benefits. Cost-utility analysis is normally used to compare the cost effectiveness of interventions in one illness with that in other illnesses so that total healthcare resources can be allocated in such a way as to optimize the total health gain from a specified budget. Comparison across a wide number of different illnesses is facilitated by the use of a common currency for the benefits of treatment, called the QALY, a quality adjusted life year gained. Results are described in terms of the additional cost required to gain a QALY.

These forms of economic evaluations have been reported in the still relatively limited but growing international literature on the economics of managing haemostasis in individuals with inhibitors.

Search Details

To compile this review, the author searched Medline and NHS CRD databases and hand reviewed abstracts from the World Federation of Hemophilia meeting (July 2000). Most publications identified examine cost of treatment only. The majority of the published full economic evaluations compare costs and benefits of activated prothrombin complex concentrate (aPCC, FEIBA) and recombinant activated coagulation factor VII (rFVIIa, NovoSeven).

Cost of Illness Studies

Cost of illness evaluations have been conducted for patients with inhibitors in a number of European countries including, France [3, 4] and Italy [5]. Their results highlight the burden haemophilia with inhibitors places on the healthcare system and on the patient. Figure 1 summarizes the results from the French study that compared the cost of managing adult patients without inhibitors (0inh, n = 103), with low responding inhibitors (LR, n = 24) and high responding inhibitors (HR, n = 17). between 1988 and 1998 during two periods: 1988–1995 and 1996–1998, before and after the introduction of rFVIIa in France (1996) [4]. In both periods, the mean cost of managing of patients with high responding inhibitors (HR) was considerably higher than that for patients with no inhibitors (0inh) and low responding inhibitors (LR). In the period 1988–95, hospitalisations and deaths

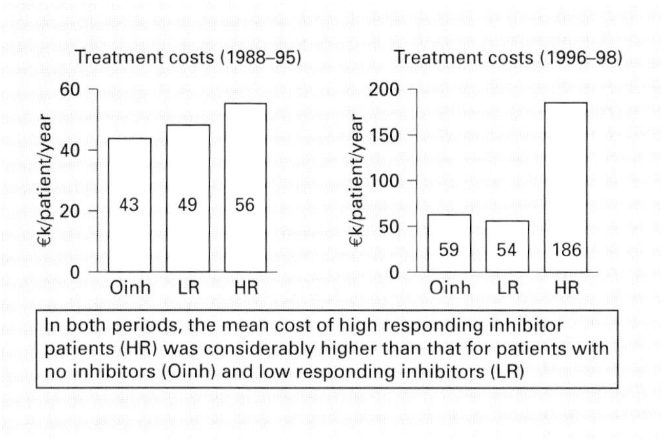

Fig. 1. Burden is greater in haemophilia patients with inhibitors: French study [4].

due to uncontrolled bleeds were more frequent in patients with high responding inhibitors than the other groups. Use of rFVIIa contributed to the increased cost in the period 1996–1998. However, the authors point out that rFVIIa was used in spontaneous severe bleeds, which in the past would not have been controlled and led to death. In addition, rFVIIa was used in eight surgical procedures that would not have been undertaken in its absence.

The Cost of Home versus Hospital Treatment in Severe Haemophilia Patients with Inhibitors

A recent case report of the economics of implementing a home treatment protocol with rFVIIa for a particularly severe inhibitor patient showed that over a 2 year period, rFVIIa was associated with lower overall treatment costs than in the 2 years previously during which the patients received aPCC (FEIBA) [6]. Whilst on rFVIIa the patient experienced considerably fewer days in hospital, suggesting better control of haemostasis.

Long Term Costs of Using rFVIIa in Surgery

As indicated in the French COI study [4], there is increased interest in the use of rFVIIa in surgery. The use of a decision analysis model to estimate the cost of haemostasis (with rFVIIa treatment) in patients undergoing surgical procedures in the UK and predict the costs of managing bleeds in these patients for 5 years post treatment has recently been published [7]. For a person weighing 75 kg , experiencing 1 bleed per month in the affected joint, the costs for haemostasis associated with total hip replacement were estimated to be £322,911. But when the reduction in future regular bleeds is accounted for, the model predicted a net saving of £298,401 over 5 years.

Can the Additional Costs be Justified by Additional Benefits?

The COI and BIA studies hinted at some of the benefits of treatment with the new haemostatic agents, however, no quantitative evaluation of benefits was carried out. The following published studies have examined the 'value for money' of these agents.

Cost Minimization Analysis in Adults with Inhibitors

Two cost minimization analyses comparing the cost of managing a minor bleed in adult inhibitor patients in hospital- [8] and home-based settings [9] using either rFVIIa or aPCC have been published. Based on a decision analysis model that described the management of bleeds using either drug, both analyses showed that in the 1st line treatment of bleeds, rFVIIa is less costly than aPCC. In addition, using rFVIIa as the initial treatment, instead of aPCC, is expected to resolve a minor bleeding episode in about half the time (30 versus 58 h). However, a major limitation of the analyses was the absence of randomized control trial data comparing the two products, necessitating the data required for the decision analysis model (describing the management of bleeds using either drug) to be taken from historical published efficacy data on both drugs, supplemented with information from a panel of haematologists.

Cost Utility Analysis in Children with Inhibitors

A cost utility analysis has been reported examining the cost-effectiveness of rFVIIa in six Australian children with long standing inhibitors to factor VIII or IX compared with usual treatment [10] (fig. 2). Using validated questionnaires, the quality of life and utility was measured in addition to medical resource use and associated costs for 3 phases: 6 months prior to rFVIIa (phase 1), first

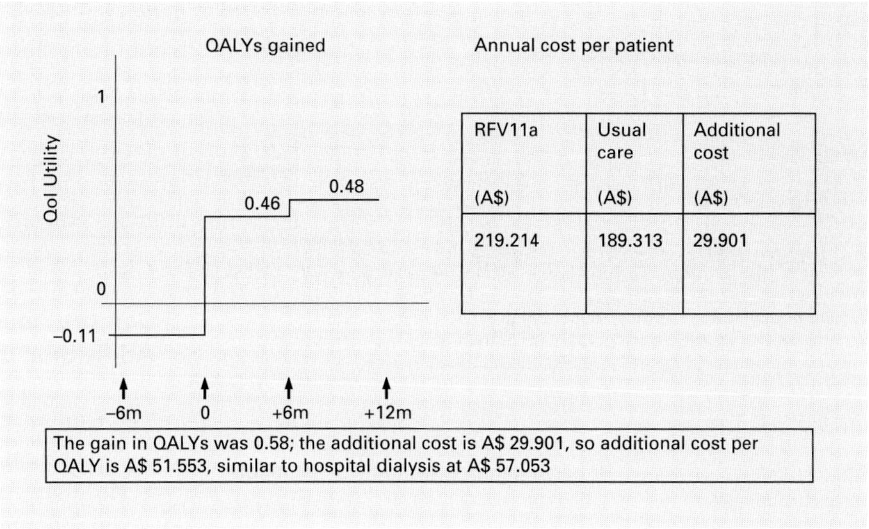

Fig. 2. Cost per QALY gained for one year of rFVIIa vs. 'usual treatment' in Australia [10].

6 months of rFVIIa and second six months of rFVIIa treatment. Patient Qol and utility improved significantly on treatment with rFVIIa, resulting in an average gain of 0.58 QALY. The additional cost per QALY gained was A$ 51,553 which is comparable with that derived for currently reimbursed healthcare strategies, including hospital dialysis (i.e. $ 57,053).

Future Research

As rFVIIa accelerates the resolution of bleeding, future research could expand our understanding of the impact of accelerated bleed resolution on long-term sequelae, including need for surgery and quality of life. The availability of a disease specific Qol instrument would be useful in this regard.

References

1 Trueman P, Drummond M, Hutton J: Developing Guidance for Budget Impact Analysis. Pharmacoeconomics 2001;19:609–621.
2 Mauskopf JE, Paul JE, Grant DM, Stergachis A: The role of cost consequence analysis in healthcare decision-making. Pharmacoeconomics 1998;13:277–288.
3 Goudemand J: Pharmaco-economic aspects of inhibitor treatment. Eur J Haematol 1998; 61(suppl 63):24–27.
4 Goudemand J: Treatment of patients with inhibitors: Cost issues. Haemophilia 1999;5: 397–401.
5 Gringeri A, Mantovani G, Santagostino E et al: COCIS (cost of care inhibitor study): Evaluation of the socio-economic impact of inhibitors in haemophiliacs. Presented at the World Federation of Hemophilia MTG, July 2000. Haemophilia 2000;6:441.
6 Stewart AJ, Hanley JP, Ludlam CA: Safety, efficacy and cost-effectiveness of home therapy with recombinant activated factor VII in a patient with severe haemophilia A and an anti-factor VIII inhibitor. Blood Coagulation and Fibrinolysis 1998;9(suppl 1):593–595.
7 Green C, de Cock E: Cost-Consequences of orthopaedic surgery in haemophilia patients with inhibitors. Abstract submitted to ISPOR (November, 2001, Cannes) and accepted for poster presentation 2001.
8 Odeyemi IAO, Guest JF: Economic impact of recombinant activated factor VII compared to activated prothrombin-complex concentrate in the hospital treatment of a mild to moderate bleed among adult haemophilia patients with inhibitors in the UK. Pharmacoeconomics 2001, in press.
9 Odeyemi IAO, Guest JF: Economic impact of recombinant activated factor VII compared with activated prothrombin-complex concentrate in the home treatment of minor bleed in adult haemophilia patients with high titre high responding inhibitors to coagulation factors VIII and IX. Presented at the 2000 Annual Meeting of the American Society of Hematology, San Francisco, Dec 2000 (abstract).
10 Ekert H, Brewin T, Boey W, Davey P, Tilden D: Cost-utility analysis of recombinant factor VIIa (NovoSeven) in six children with long-standing inhibitors to factor VIII or IX. Haemophilia 2001;7:279–285.

Pathophysiology of Haemostasis and Thrombosis

Pathophysiol Haemost Thromb 2002;32(suppl 1):33–36

General Haemostatic Agents – Fact or Fiction?

Ulla Hedner

Novo Nordisk A/S, Copenhagen, Denmark

Key Words
Haemostasis failure · Thrombin · rFVIIa

Abstract
Haemophilia is the most serious bleeding model that nature has provided us with, indicating the importance of factor FVIII and FIX in haemostasis. According to current knowledge, haemostasis is initiated by the formation of a complex between tissue factor (TF), exposed as a result of a vessel wall injury, and activated FVII (FVIIa) that is normally present in circulating blood. The TF-FVIIa complexes convert FX into FXa on the TF-bearing cell. FXa then activates prothrombin into thrombin. This limited amount of thrombin activates FVIII, FV, FXI and platelets. Thrombin-activated platelets change shape, resulting in exposure of negatively-charged phospholipids, which form the perfect template for full thrombin generation involving FVIII and FIX. In patients with haemophilia FVIII or FIX is missing. These individuals generate only initial limited amounts of thrombin as its generation is dependent on the presence of FVIII and FIX. Full thrombin generation is necessary for complete activation of FXIII and thrombin activatable fibrinolytic inhibitor to occur. Furthermore, full thrombin generation is important for the fibrin structure of the haemostatic plug. In the case of impaired thrombin generation, fibrin plugs will be loose and highly permeable. Such fibrin plugs are easily dissolved by normal fibrinolytic activity and thus prevent full and maintained haemostasis from occurring. The addition of rFVIIa to FVIII- or FIX-deficient plasma has been shown to increase thrombin generation in a cell-based in vitro model. Furthermore, extra rFVIIa was found to normalise fibrin clot permeability in vitro and to tighten the fibrin structure as studied by three-dimensional confocal microscopy. These findings indicate that administration of rFVIIa is capable of compensating for the lack of FVIII and FIX. Accordingly, the administration of exogenous rFVIIa has been found to stop bleedings in haemophilia patients and, provided it is given in doses high enough, to allow major surgery to be performed in severe haemophiliacs with inhibitors. As rFVIIa enhances thrombin generation on already activated platelets, it has been suggested that rFVIIa may also help to improve haemostasis in other situations involving impaired thrombin generation, such as platelet disorders (thrombocytopenia and functional platelet defects). Preliminary clinical data appear to support this. Patients with profuse bleeding due to extensive surgery or trauma often develop a complex coagulation pattern which includes reduced plasma levels of fibrinogen, FVIII and FV, and decreased platelet counts. These patients may

KARGER
Fax + 41 61 306 12 34
E-Mail karger@karger.ch
www.karger.com

1424–8832/02/0327–0033$18.50/0

Accessible online at:
www.karger.com/journals/pht

Prof. Ulla Hedner
Novo Nordisk A/S, Carlsgatan 19
S–21618 Malmo (Sweden)
Tel. +46 40 162869, Fax +46 40 162819, E-Mail uhe@novonordisk.com

well have an impaired capacity to generate thrombin. Consequently, they may benefit from one or two doses of rFVIIa in order to assist in the generation of a thrombin peak sufficient to form a firm, stable fibrin haemostatic plug and thereby reduce bleeding. This would facilitate any mechanical repair necessary for full haemostasis. Preliminary results in a few patients may support such an effect for rFVIIa. As thrombin has such a crucial role in providing haemostasis, any agent that enhances the thrombin generation in situations with an impaired thrombin formation may be characterised as a 'general haemostatic agent'. Let us look forward to more 'facts' through the 'evidence-based route'.

Introduction

Failure of haemostasis is one of the most ominous events in clinical medicine. For the surgeon, it is potentially catastrophic and a number of haemostatic agents for topical use have been developed over the years. Haemostasis is the cumulative effect occurring as a result of many events. The vessels, platelets, the coagulation and the fibrinolytic systems are all involved. Defective platelets as well as lowered platelet counts result in an impaired thrombin generation and so does a defective coagulation system. Thrombin is necessary for haemostasis by converting the soluble fibrinogen into fibrin.

A number of agents are being used to achieve haemostasis. Such agents may be used topically or systemically. Topical haemostatic agents include vasoconstrictive agents such as epinephrine and procoagulant agents such as thrombin, 'haemostatic fibrin', gelatin, cellulose material for example spongostan. Systemically administered haemostatic agents include coagulation factors which can be used in situations of vitamin K deficiency where the vitamin K-dependent factors are low. The thrombin used so far is, however, bovine and development of cross-reacting antibodies against prothrombin and other coagulation proteins such as FV present in the thrombin solution have been reported [1, 2]. 'Haemostatic fibrin' also contains other coagulation proteins of bovine origin which may initiate the formation of cross-reacting antibodies. The use of gelatin and cellulose material are often restricted depending on clinical settings. A general haemostatic agent may be one that enhances full thrombin generation and thereby the formation of a stabile, tight fibrin haemostatic plug resistant to premature fibrinolysis.

Normal Haemostasis

According to current knowledge haemostasis is initiated by the formation of a complex between tissue factor (TF) exposed as a result of a vessel wall injury, and already activated FVII (FVIIa) normally present in the circulating blood in a concentration corresponding to about 1% of the total FVII protein mass [3]. The TF-FVIIa complexes convert FX into FXa on the TF bearing cell. FXa then activates prothrombin into thrombin [4, 5]. This limited amount of thrombin activates FVIII, FV, FXI and platelets. Thrombin-activated platelets change shape and as a result will expose negatively charged phospholipids, which form the perfect template for full thrombin generation involving FVIII and FIX. Thrombin also converts the soluble fibrinogen into fibrin, it activates FXIII, the fibrin stabilizing enzyme, as well as the thrombin activatable fibrinolytic inhibitor (TAFI). The fibrin structure has been found to be dependent on the amount of thrombin formed and the rate of thrombin generation [6].

In summary, full generation of thrombin is necessary for the formation of a tight, stabile fibrin haemostatic plug resistant to premature fibrinolysis, which is required for full and sustained haemostasis.

Recombinant FVIIa in Patients with an Impaired Thrombin Generation

Haemophilia

Haemophilia is the most serious bleeding model nature has provided us with. Patients with haemophilia lack FVIII or FIX and therefore, haemophilia patients only generate the initial limited amounts of thrombin and never get the full thrombin generation which is dependent on the presence of FVIII and FIX [7]. Recently, it was demonstrated that thrombin is generated on the surface of thrombin activated platelets in the absence of FIX provided extra FVIIa is added. Concentrations of FVIIa of at least 50 n*M* are required to achieve thrombin amounts in the area of what is seen in the presence of FVIII/FIX [8, 9]. The FVIIa binding to the activated platelets is a low affinity binding and therefore, the amounts necessary for thrombin generation is many fold higher than the concentration of FVIIa normally present in the blood (0.2 n*M*). Using the same cell-based model as being used by Monroe et al., a dose response of the thrombin generation following the addition of increasing concentrations of rFVIIa was demonstrated [10]. Concentrations of rFVIIa of up to 150 n*M* were required to achieve a similar thrombin generation as seen in the presence of FVIII and FIX (in the absence of FXI). Furthermore, extra rFVIIa was found to normalize the fibrin clot permeability in vitro and to tighten the fibrin structure as studied by 3D confocal microscopy [11]. This would indicate that the administration of extra rFVIIa is capable of compensating for the lack of FVIII and FIX in the generation of a full thrombin generation and the formation of tight fibrin plugs resistant to premature lysis thereby initiating full and sustained haemostasis.

Accordingly, the administration of exogenous rFVIIa has been found to stop bleedings in haemophilia patients and, provided it is given in doses high enough, to allow major surgery in severe haemophiliacs with inhibitors [12].

Other Situations Characterized by Impaired Thrombin Generation

Based on the in vitro data indicating that rFVIIa enhances thrombin generation and thereby results in the formation of tight, and less porous fibrin structure, it may be hypothesized that the addition of extra rFVIIa may be beneficial in other situations than haemophilia with impaired thrombin generation. Defective thrombin generation is known to occur in patients with thrombocytopenia as well as in patients with functionally defective platelets [13]. Also, thrombin generation in the cell-based model was demonstrated to be dependent on the number of platelets present. Furthermore, the lag phase of the platelet activation was found to shorten in a dose-dependent manner after the addition of rFVIIa in the same model [14]. However, the thrombin peak did not normalize as a result of the added rFVIIa. It has, however, been stressed by Blombäck et al [6] that not only the amount of thrombin but the rate of thrombin generation are also important for the formation of a tight fibrin structure. Preliminary clinical data seem to support a beneficial effect of extra rFVIIa in patients with bleedings and defective platelets [15, 16].

Potentially impaired thrombin generation may be involved in patients with a complex coagulation pattern as a result of massive bleedings in association with extensive surgery or trauma. Such patients often have lowered plasma levels of a number of various coagulation proteins such as fibrinogen, FVIII, FV etc. In addition, thrombocytopenia is common as well as an increased fibrinolysis as a result of massive tissue damage. Several of these factors are important for an adequate thrombin formation as well as for the formation of a tight fibrin plug. Thus, low levels of fibrinogen result in the formation of a loose fibrin structure and to a decreased activation of FXIII, the fibrin stabilizing factor [17]. These patients thus may benefit from one or two doses of rFVIIa in order to help to generate a thrombin peak, which may be enough to form a firm, stable fibrin haemostatic plug and thereby decrease the bleeding [9]. This would facilitate any mechanical repair necessary for full haemostasis. Preliminary results in a few patients may support such an effect of extra rFVIIa [18, 19].

Since thrombin has such a crucial role in providing haemostasis, any agent that enhances thrombin generation in situations with impaired thrombin formation may be characterized as a 'general haemostatic agent'.

References

1 Berruyer M, Amiral J, Ffrench P, Belleville J, Bastien O, Clerc J, Kassir A, Estanove S, Dechavanne M: Immunization by bovine thrombin used with fibrin glue during cardiovascular operations. Development of thrombin and factor V inhibitors. J Thorac Cardiovasc Surg 1993;105:892–897.

2 Chouhan VD, De La C, Nagaswami C, Weisel JW, Kajani M, Rao AK: Simultaneous occurrence of human antibodies directed against fibrinogen, thrombin, and factor V following exposure to bovine thrombin: Effects on blood coagulation, protein C activation and platelet function. Thromb Haemost 1997;77:343–349.

3 Wildgoose P, Nemerson Y, Hansen LL, Nielsen FE, Glazer S, Hedner U: Measurement of basal levels of factor VIIa in hemophilia A and B patients. Blood 1992;80:25–28.

4 Rapaport SI, Rao LV: Initiation and regulation of tissue factor-dependent blood coagulation. Arterioscler Thromb 1992;12:1111–1121.

5 Rapaport SI, Rao LV: The tissue factor pathway: How it has become a 'prima ballerina'. Thromb Haemost 1995;74:7–17.

6 Blomback B, Carlsson K, Fatah K, Hessel B, Procyk R: Fibrin in human plasma: Gel architectures governed by rate and nature of fibrinogen activation. Thromb Res 1994;75:521–538.

7 Hoffman M, Monroe DM, Oliver JA, Roberts HR: Factors IXa and Xa play distinct roles in tissue factor-dependent initiation of coagulation. Blood 1995;86:1794–1801.

8 Monroe DM, Hoffman M, Oliver JA, Roberts HR: Platelet activity of high-dose factor VIIa is independent of tissue factor. Brit J Haematol 1997;99:542–547.

9 Hedner U: NovoSeven as a Universal haemostatic agent. Blood Coagulation Fibrinolysis 2000;11(suppl 1):107–111.

10 Kjalke M, Ezban M, Hedner U: Increased initial thrombin generation may explain the efficacy of high-dose factor VIIa in thrombocytopenia. Blood 1999;94:451a.

11 He S, Blomback M, Hedner U: Effect of rFVIIa on the permeability of fibrin gel. Thromb Haemost 2001;CD3315 (abstract).
12 Shapiro AD, Gilchrist GS, Hoots WK, Cooper HA, Gastineau DA: Prospective, randomised trial of two doses of rFVIIa (NovoSeven) in haemophilia patients with inhibitors undergoing surgery. Thromb Haemost 1998;80:773–778.
13 Keularts IM, Beguin S, de Zwaan C, Hemker HC: Treatment with a GPIIb/IIIa antagonist inhibits thrombin generation in platelet rich plasma from patients. Thromb Haemost 1998; 80:370–371.
14 Kjalke M, Ezban M, Monroe DM, Hoffman M, Roberts HR, Hedner U: High-dose factor VIIa increases initial thrombin generation and mediates faster platelet activation in thrombocytopenia-like conditions in a cell-based model system. Br J Haematol 2001;114:114–120.
15 Kristensen J, Killander A, Hippe E, Helleberg C, Ellegard J, Holm M, Kutti J, Mellqvist UH, Johansson JE, Glazer S, Hedner U: Clinical experience with recombinant factor VIIa in patients with thrombocytopenia. Haemostasis 1996;26(suppl 1):159–164.
16 Poon MC, Demers C, Jobin F, Wu JW: Recombinant factor VIIa is effective for bleeding and surgery in patients with Glanzmann thrombasthenia. Blood 1999;94:3951–3953.
17 McDonagh J, Fukue H: Determinants of substrate specificity for factor XIII. Semin Thromb Hemost 1996;22:369–376.
18 Kenet G, Walden R, Eldad A, Martinowitz U: Treatment of traumatic bleeding with recombinant factor VIIa. Lancet 1999;354:1879.
19 Martinowitz U, Holcomb JB, Pusateri AE, Stein M, Onaca N, Freidman M, Macaitis JM, Castel D, Hedner U, Hess JR: Intravenous rFVIIa administered for hemorrhage control in hypothermic coagulopathic swine with grade V liver injuries. J Trauma 2001;50:721–729.

Pathophysiology of Haemostasis and Thrombosis

Pathophysiol Haemost Thromb 2002;32(suppl 1):37–40

Treatment of Bleeding in Patients with Platelet Disorders: Is There a Place for Recombinant Factor VIIa?

Yves Laurian

Novo Nordisk Pharmaceutique SA, Boulogne-Billancourt, France

Key Words
Thrombocytopenia · Inherited thrombocytopathia · Glanzmann thrombasthenia · Bleeding · rFVIIa

Abstract
The mechanism of action of recombinant factor VIIa (rFVIIa), i.e. increased thrombin generation on the membrane of activated platelets, as well as the results from in vitro and ex vivo models of thrombocytopenia or inherited thrombocytopathia may support some potential of rFVIIa in thrombocytopenia/thrombocytopathia. rFVIIa was reported as effective to stop or to decrease bleeding in few patients with severe thrombocytopenia resistant to platelet transfusions; however data are still scarce and clinical studies are really needed to define efficacy/safety ratio as well as optimal treatment regimen in this potential indication. Some data in patients with Glanzmann thrombasthenia (GT) may support the use of rFVIIa outside its primary indication in the cases in which there is no real treatment alternative (GT patients with antibodies to GP IIb-IIIa or with platelet refractoriness).

Introduction

Recombinant factor VIIa (rFVIIa; NovoSeven®) was approved for the treatment of bleeding episodes and the prevention of bleeding during surgery in patients with haemophilia and inhibitors and in patients with acquired haemophilia [1–5]. In this indication, rFVIIa demonstrated an excellent efficacy and safety profile [6, 7]. rFVIIa is produced without any human derivatives (no risk of transmission of viruses or other transmissible agents from human origin; no risk of anamnestic rise of the inhibitor titre) [1, 5]. Optimal results were observed when rFVIIa is used as first-line therapy [4, 8, 9] and with optimal treatment regimen [1–3].

Mode of Action

The proposed mechanism of action of rFVIIa in patients with haemophilia is an increased thrombin generation on the membrane of the activated platelets localized at the site of bleeding [10–12] allowing a better fibrin clot less prone to fibrinolysis and a better activation of factor XIII and of thrombin activable fibrinolysis inhibitor (TAFI). Decreased thrombin generation was previously reported in patients with thrombocytopenia, with Glanzmann thrombasthenia (GT) and with Bernard-Soulier

KARGER
Fax + 41 61 306 12 34
E-Mail karger@karger.ch
www.karger.com

1424–8832/02/0327–0037$18.50/0

Accessible online at:
www.karger.com/journals/pht

Yves Laurian, MD
Novo Nordisk Pharmaceutique SA
32, rue de Bellevue
F–92273 Boulogne-Billancourt (France)
Fax +33 1 46 84 59 53, E-Mail yvla@novonordisk.com

syndrome (BSS). This raises the question whether rFVIIa could be a potential candidate as a new haemostatic drug for bleeding in these patients. Some in vitro/ex vivo data [13–14] as well as some case reports [15, 16] may support rFVIIa as a drug with potentiality in platelet disorders.

Thrombocytopenia

High dose of recombinant factor VIIa was reported

- to shorten significantly the microvascular bleeding time in thrombocytopenic rabbits
- to increase the initial thrombin generation, resulting in faster platelet activation in an in vitro model of severe thrombocytopenia [13]
- to enhance fibrin deposition in a chamber under flow conditions using thrombocytopenic blood [14].

However, high dose of rFVIIa did not increase, in the in vitro model of thrombocytopenia, the rate of thrombin generation which remains very low when compared to normal [13] and there was no improvement of platelet deposition on subendothelium under flow conditions [14].

A study was undertaken in 74 patients with moderate to severe thrombocytopenia related to either impaired platelet production or immune destruction to evaluate the safety of rFVIIa in patients with thrombocytopenia but normal coagulation factors [15]. Each patient received a single dose of 50 and/or 100 μg/kg. A total of 111 injections were given. The clinical tolerance was excellent, except one anaphylactoid reaction in a patient with previous history of such reactions with other drugs. A reduction of the bleeding time was found in 55/105 cases after a single dose of rFVIIa (50 or 100 μg/kg). This reduction was significantly more pronounced when the platelet count exceeded $20 \times 10^9/l$. However, these results must be discussed with caution since no venostasis pressure was applied in patients with impaired platelet production (47 patients; 66 cases). Ten minor/moderate bleeds (neck incision, epistaxis, uterine bleed) were treated with a single dose of rFVIIa (50 or 100 μg/kg) in 8 patients with moderate to severe thrombocytopenia (3 patients with platelets $\leq 10 \times 10^9/l$; 3 patients with 11–20 and 2 patients >20–33) [15]. Bleeding stopped in 7 cases and slowed down or almost ceased in the last 3 cases. There was no clear correlation between shortening of bleeding time and stop of bleeding. Since then no result of clinical trials have been published. Only case stories have appeared in the literature [17, 18].

rFVIIa has some potential in thrombocytopenia, but many questions remain unsolved:

- Efficacy/safety ratio and cost-effectiveness?
- Minimal number of platelets required to get efficacy of rFVIIa?
- Treatment regimen (dose of rFVIIa per injection; number of doses to stop the bleed; interval between doses)?
- Need for additional doses to avoid recurrence of bleeding when stopped?
- Use of rFVIIa alone or in addition to platelets transfusion when very low platelet count?
- Benefit of addition of platelets transfusion in case of complete platelet refractoriness with no circulating platelets?

Only a full clinical development with randomised studies may answer these questions and allow to evaluate the possible place of rFVIIa in patients with bleeding related to severe thrombocytopenia.

Inherited Thrombocytopathia

Inherited platelet function disorders with bleeding tendency are very rare, including Glanzmann thrombasthenia (GT), Bernard-Soulier syndrome (BSS), pseudo-Willebrand and few other diseases [5]. The treatment of bleeding or prevention of bleeding for surgery/invasive procedure is based on platelet transfusion when local measures and antifibrinolytic drug failed. However platelet transfusions may be responsible for development of antibodies to GP IIb-IIIa, GP Ib or HLA with high-risk of future platelet refractoriness [19, 20]. Moreover platelet concentrates have a low but real residual risk of viral contamination.

Decreased thrombin generation was previously reported in patients with GT and in patients with BSS. rFVIIa was reported to increase local fibrin deposition as well as partially restore platelet aggregates in GLZ as well as in BSS [14]. These data may support rFVIIa as a potential haemostatic candidate in these patients.

rFVIIa was reported to stop or prevent bleeding in patients with GLZ with or without antibody to GP IIb-IIIa [16, 19–27]. The result of a pilot study was published [19] on the use of rFVIIa to treat 24 bleeding episodes and to prevent bleeding during one bilateral herniorrhaphy in 4 patients with GT. rFVIIa was administered at 89 to 116 μg/kg per injection every 2 h, in association with antifibrinolytic drugs. Bleeding stopped with rFVIIa in all, but one case and there was no abnormal bleeding during and after the surgical procedure. In two cases, the bleeding recurred 36 and 63 h after discontinuation of rFVIIa, but the two episodes were successfully treated with additional doses of rFVIIa. Data on the use of rFVIIa in patients with GLZ were collected in an international data collection [26, 27]. In the last presentation of these data [27], intention to treat analysis with rFVIIa showed efficacy in all 11 evaluable invasive/surgical procedures and in 73% of the 55 bleeding episodes (fig. 1).

Taking into account these data [16, 19–27], rFVIIa may be particularly helpful in GT patients with antibodies to GP IIb-IIIa or to HLA or in patients with platelet inefficacy, since treatment alternatives are scarce and may not be efficacious [19, 20, 26, 27].

In other inherited thrombocytopathia, a single patient with BSS [28] and one with pseudo von Willebrand disease [29] were reported to be treated efficiently with rFVIIa.

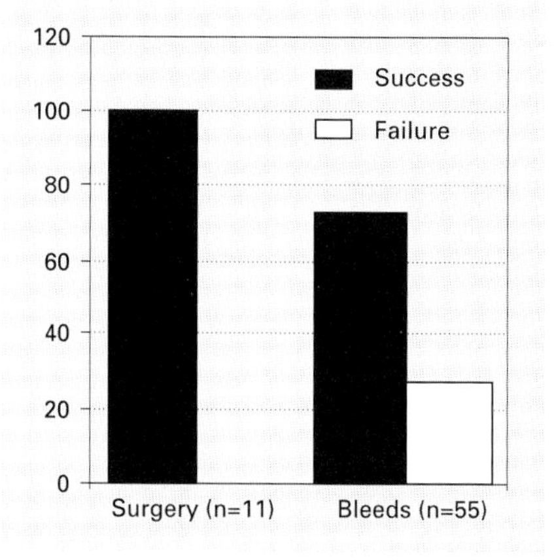

Fig. 1. Intention to treat with recombinant factor VIIa in patients with Glanzmann thrombasthenia.

Acquired Thrombocytopathia

Recombinant FVIIa was reported as efficient for few bleeds related to uremic syndrome [30, 31] and to acquired thrombocytopathia related to myelodysplasic syndrome [32], but no other data have been yet published in peer-reviewed paper on acquired thrombocytopathia.

Discussion

rFVIIa is a drug with real potentiality in platelet disorders. Clinical data may support the use of rFVIIa, outside its primary indication, in GT patients with antibodies to GP IIb-IIIa or to HLA or with platelet inefficacy due to the absence of real alternative treatment [19, 20, 22, 26, 27]. For patients with thrombocytopenia, clinical data are still too scarce and there is a major need for full clinical development, including randomised double-blind study whenever possible, to demonstrate efficacy and safety of rFVIIa as well as cost-efficacy. Clinical development was recently started. While awaiting the results of such studies, some question the use of rFVIIa outside its indication in cases of persistent life-threatening bleeds despite adequate platelet transfusions [17, 18]; however there is no data yet to support any treatment regimen as well as the use or not of concomitant platelet transfusions.

References

1 Hedner U: NovoSeven® as a universal hemostatic agent. Blood Coagul Fibrinolysis 2000;11(suppl 1):S107–S111.
2 Shapiro A, Gilchrist GS, Hoots WK, Cooper HA, Gastineau DA: Prospective, randomised trial of two doses of rFVIIa (Novoseven) in haemophilia patients with inhibitors undergoing Surgery. Thromb Haemost 1998;80:773–778.
3 Key NS, Aledort LM, Beardsley D, Cooper HA, Davignon G, Ewenstein BM, Gilchrist GS, Gill JC, Glader B, Hoots WK, Kisker CT, Lusher JM, Rosenfield CG, Shapiro AD, Smith H, Taft E: Home treatment of mild to moderate bleeding episodes using recombinant factor VIIa (NovoSeven) in haemophiliacs with inhibitors. Thromb Haemost 1998;80:912–918.
4 Hay CRM, Negrier C, Ludlam CA: The treatment of bleeding in acquired haemophilia with recombinant factor VIIa: A multicentre study. Thromb Haemost 1997;78:1463–1467.
5 Poon M.C: Use of recombinant factor VIIa in hereditary bleeding disorders. Curr Opin Hematol 2001;8:312–318.
6 Roberts HR: Clinical experience with activated factor VII: focus on safety aspects. Blood Coagul Fibrinolysis 1998;9(suppl 1):S115–S118.
7 Aledort LM: Recombinant factor VIIa is a panhemostatic agent. Thromb Haemost 2000;83:637–638.
8 Lusher JM: Acute hemarthroses: the benefits of early versus late treatment with recombinant activated factor VII. Blood Coagul Fibrinolysis 2000;11(suppl 1):S45–S48.
9 Lusher JM: Recombinant activated factor VII for treatment of intramuscular haemorrhages: A comparison of early versus late treatment. Blood Coagul Fibrinolysis 1998;9(suppl 1):S111–S114.
10 Monroe DM, Hoffman M, Oliver JA, Roberts HR: Platelet activity of high-dose factor VIIa is independent of tissue factor. Br J Haematol 1997;99:542–547.
11 Hoffmann M, Monroe DM, Roberts HR: Activated factor VII activates factors IX and X on the surface of activated platelets: Thoughts on the mechanism of action of high-dose activated factor VII. Blood Coagul Fibrinolysis 1998;9(suppl 1):S61–S65.

12 Hoffman M, Monroe DM: A cell-based model of hemostasis. Thromb Haemost 2001;85:958–965.
13 Kjalke M, Ezban M, Monroe DM, Hoffmann M, Roberts HR, Hedner U: High-dose factor VIIa increases initial thrombin generation and mediates faster platelet activation in thrombocytopenia-like conditions in a cell-based model system. Br J Haematol 2001;114:114–120.
14 Galan M, Reverter JC, Pino M, Vinas M, Lozano M, Ordinas A, Escolar G: Increased local procoagulant action: A mechanism contributing to the favourable hemostatic effect of activated recombinant factor VII (rFVIIa) in quanti- and qualitative disorders of platelet function. XVIII Congress of the International Society of Thrombosis and Haemostasis, Paris, France, 6–12 July 2001 (abstract).
15 Kristensen J, Killander A, Hippe E, Helleberg C, Ellegard J, Holm M, Kutti J, Mellqvist UH, Johansson JE, Glazer S, Hedner U: Clinical experience with recombinant factor VIIa in patients with thrombocytopenia. Haemostasis 1996;26(suppl 1):159–164.
16 Tengborn L, Petruson B: A patient with Glanzmann thrombasthenia and epistaxis successfully treated with recombinant factor VII. Thromb Haemost 1996;75:981–982.
17 Vidarsson B, Önundarson PT: Recombinant factor VIIa for bleeding in refractory thrombocytopenia. Thromb Haemost 2000;83:634–635.
18 Blatt J, Gold SH, Wiley JM, Monahan PE, Cooper HC, Harvey D: Off-label use of recombinant factor VIIa in patients following bone marrow transplantation. Bone Marrow Transplantation 2001;28:405–407.
19 Poon M-C, Demers C, Jobin F, Wu JWY: Recombinant factor VIIa is effective for bleeding and surgery in patients with Glanzmann thrombasthenia. Blood 1999;94:3951–3953.
20 d'Oiron R, Ménart C, Trzeciak C, Nurden P, Fressinaud E, Dreyfus M, Laurian Y, Négrier C: Use of recombinant factor VIIa in 3 patients with inherited type I Glanzmann's thrombasthenia undergoing invasive procedures. Thromb Haemost 2000;83:644–647.
21 Wielenga JJ, Siebel Y, van Buuren HR, Berends FJ, Schipperus MER, van Vliet HDDM, Kappers MC: Use of recombinant factor VIIa and HLA matched platelets to prevent bleeding during and after major surgery in a patient with Glanzmann thromboasthenia. Haemophilia 1998;4: XXIIIth Congress of the World Federation of Hemophilia (abstract).
22 Patel RK, Savidge GF, Rangarajan S: Use of recombinant factor VIIa for post-operative haemorrhage in a patient with Glanzmann's thrombasthenia and human leucocyte antigen antibodies. Br J Haematol 2001;114:245–246.
23 Ancliff P, Liesner R, Khair K, Hann I: The use of recombinant factor VIIa in a patient with severe Glanzmann's thrombasthenia to facilitate insertion of a Port-a-Cath®. Blood Coagul Fibrinolysis 1999;10:447–448.
24 Chuansumrit A, Sangkapreecha C, Hathirat P. Successful epistaxis control in a patient with Glanzmann thrombasthenia by increased bolus injection dose of recombinant factor VIIa. Thromb Haemost 1999;82:1178.
25 Musso R, Cultrera D, Russo M, Giuffrida G, Venturino L, Ferlito C, Salerni S, Azzaro MP, Incatasciato D: Recombinant activated factor VII as haemostatic agent in Glanzmann's thromboastenia. Thromb Haemost 1999 (suppl), XVIIth Congress of the International Society on Thrombosis and Haemostasis (abstract).
26 Poon MC, d'Oiron R & the International Registry on Recombinant Factor VIIa and Congenital Platelet Disorders Group Recombinant activated factor VII (Novoseven®) in the treatment of platelet-related bleeding disorders. Blood Coagul Fibrinolysis 2000;11(suppl 1): S55–S68.
27 Poon MC, Katsarou O, Huth-Kuehne A, Petrini P, Hann I, Demers C, Fressinaud E, Tengborn L, Thomas A, Nohe N, Strauss G, Négrier C, Makris PE, Molho P, Pautard B, Berger C, Beurrier P, Wilde J, Devecioglu O, Peters M, d'Oiron R: Recombinant factor VIIa in congenital platelet bleeding disordersAmerican Society of Hematology 2000, 1–5 December, San Francisco. Blood; 96(suppl 1):256a (abstract).
28 Peters M, Heijboer H: Treatment of a patient with Bernard-Soulier syndrome and recurrent nosebleeds with recombinant factor VIIa. Thromb Haemost 1998;80:352.
29 Fressinaud E, Sigaud-Fiks M, Le Boterff C, Piot B: Use of recombinant factor VIIa (NovoSeven®) for dental extraction in a patient affected by platelet-type (pseudo-) von Willebrand disease. Haemophilia 1998;4: XXIIIth Congress of the World Federation of Hemophilia (abstract).
30 Revesz T, Arets B, Bierings M, van den Bos C, Duval E: Recombinant factor VIIa in severe uremic bleeding. Thromb Haemost 1998;80: 353.
31 Moisescu E, Ardelean L, Simion I, Muresan A, Ciupan R: Recombinant factor VIIa treatment of bleeding associated with acute renal failure. Blood Coagul Fibrinolysis 2000;11:575–577.
32 Meijer K, Sieders E, Slooff JH, de Wolf JTM, van der Meer J: Effective treatment of severe bleeding due to acquired thrombocytopathia by single dose administration of activated recombinant factor VII. Thromb Haemost 1998; 80:204–205.

Pathophysiology of Haemostasis and Thrombosis

Pathophysiol Haemost Thromb 2002;32(suppl 1):41–46

The Use of Recombinant Factor VIIa in Controlling Surgical Bleeding in Non-Haemophiliac Patients

Maadh Aldouri

Consultant Haematologist, Medway Maritime Hospital, Gillingham, UK

Key Words

Non-haemophiliac intractable bleeding · rFVIIa · Cardiac surgery · Cessation of blood loss · Trauma

Abstract

Recombinant factor VIIa (rFVIIa, NovoSeven®) is effective and appears safe in the management of bleeding episodes and provision of surgical cover in haemophilia patients with inhibitors. Additionally, rFVIIa has been considered as a universal haemostatic agent, prompting its use in the management of severe uncontrolled surgical bleeding in patients without pre-existing coagulopathies. Recombinant FVIIa has been used in 5 patients (aged 2.5 to 73.0 years; median 48 years) with uncontrolled bleeding during or after open-heart surgery. Satisfactory haemostasis was achieved with a single dose or rFVIIa 30 µg/kg, that resulted in reduction of blood loss from a mean of 4,170 ml (650–8,000 ml) to 262.5 ml (220–334 ml). No significant adverse events were reported. Recombinant FVIIa was also successfully used in controlling post-surgical bleeding in two patients with Crohn's disease, one patient with bleeding duodenal ulcer and another with false thoracic aneurysm. It was also effective in controlling bleeding post-splenectomy in a patient with chronic myeloid leukaemia, and following anterior exenteration in a patient with cervical carcinoma. A randomised study comparing the efficacy of a single perioperative dose of rFVIIa with placebo in patients undergoing transabdominal prostatectomy was conducted by Levi and colleagues [6]. An interim analysis showed a significant reduction in mean blood loss from 2,450 ± 350 ml to 1,400 ± 190 ml between placebo and rFVIIa groups respectively (p = 0.007). Among trauma patients, Kenet et al. reported success in treating uncontrolled bleeding from a gun-shot wound to the inferior vena cava, using two doses of rFVIIa 60 µg/kg [7]. This treatment has subsequently been used in 6 surgical patients with uncontrolled bleeding and in 7 cases of traumatic bleeding, with remarkable results. In conclusion, rFVIIa appears to be effective and safe in the management of uncontrolled surgical and traumatic haemorrhage in patients not known to have inherited coagulopathy.

Introduction

Over the past 13 years, rFVIIa has become established as a safe and effective treatment for haemophiliac patients with inhibitors and for other haemostatic disorders. More recently there has been a growing realisation that rFVIIa may also have a major role to play as a universal haemostatic agent. In particular, rFVIIa has been used increasingly in the treatment of non-haemophiliac patients who have severe uncontrolled bleeding associated with surgery or trauma. Although no major clinical trials have yet been carried out using rFVIIa to stem continuous bleeding in patients without coagulopathies, numerous case reports and small studies suggest that the agent brings remarkable benefits to such patients.

KARGER

Fax +41 61 306 12 34
E-Mail karger@karger.ch
www.karger.com

1424–8832/02/0327–0041$18.50/0

Accessible online at:
www.karger.com/journals/pht

Dr. Maadh Aldouri
Department of Haematology, Medway Maritime Hospital
Windmill Road, Gillingham, Kent ME7 5NY (UK)
Tel. +44 1634 825214, Fax +44 1634 825230, E-Mail mdouri@doctors.org.uk

rFVIIa in Cardiac Surgery

Cardiac surgery is often complicated by excessive blood loss. Management of the blood loss typically involves transfusion of blood components and haemostatic agents. If the bleeding continues, the patient may require a second operation and even this fails in some cases to halt the bleeding.

An investigation has been carried out by our group to see whether severe uncontrolled bleeding during cardiac surgery can be successfully treated with rFVIIa [1]. The study involved several patients undergoing open heart surgery between 1998 and1999 at the Prince Sultan Cardiac Centre in Saudi Arabia. Patients were included in this open label study if they had a blood loss of more than 150 ml/h for an average adult or more than 2 ml/kg for body weight less than 50 or more than 90 kg, for 3 consecutive hours starting 1 h postoperatively. Patients were also included if they had excessive bleeding or oozing during surgery which compromised haemodynamic stability. The patients failed to respond to adequate conventional blood components support. Patients were excluded if they had other haemostatic agents within 48 h, or a previous history of thrombosis, stroke, or ischaemic heart disease.

A dose of rFVIIa of 30 μg/kg could be given 3-hourly until bleeding was controlled, with a maximum of 4 doses.

Case 1

The first patient was a boy aged 2.5 years who had transposition of the great vessels, with a previous shunt insertion at 6 months. He underwent surgery for arterial switch with closure of the atrial septal defect and of the shunt, and construction of the pulmonary artery. This patient, who weighed 10 kg, lost 4.5 litres (l) of blood during surgery. After administration of a single dose of rFVIIa, the blood loss fell suddenly and dramatically to 30 ml in the first hour following the injection (fig. 1).

Case 2

A 73-year-old woman suffering from rheumatic heart disease and triple valve disease with heart failure and impaired left ventricular ejection fraction, underwent mitral valve replacement and tricuspid valve repair. She lost 700 ml/h of blood post-operatively, and had a second operation during which 1,900 ml of blood was drained. After the second surgery, she lost 2.7 l of blood over 3 h. An injection of rFVIIa immediately resulted in diminution of the blood loss, which fell to 80 ml during the first hour following the dose of rFVIIa (fig. 2).

Case 3

The third patient was a 48-year-old woman with complex rheumatic heart disease with heart failure, who required two valve replacements. Post-operatively, her blood loss was 500 ml/h. She had a second operation for insertion of a right ventricular assist device and intra-aortic balloon pump, after which she continued to lose blood at up to 300 ml/h. She received rFVIIa 3 h after the second operation, and her blood loss fell to 90 ml/h during the next hour (fig. 3). This patient died 3 days later; this was due to heart failure, not to blood loss.

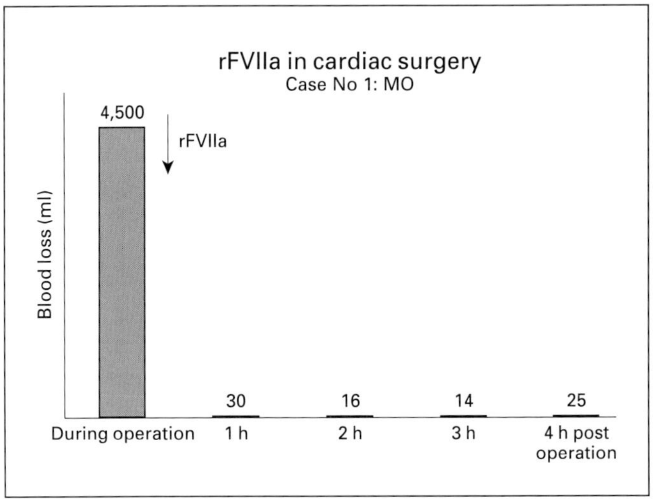

Fig. 1. rFVIIa in cardiac surgery – case No. 1: MO: Reduction in blood loss following rFVIIa administration in a 2.5-year-old boy undergoing surgery for arterial switch and pulmonary artery reconstruction [1].

Case 4

A 66-year-old man with rheumatic heart disease and heart failure underwent aortic valve repair. He had 5 l of blood loss interoperatively. A single dose of rFVIIa reduced the loss to 80 ml/h during the next hour (fig. 4).

Case 5

A 48-year-old man with mitral valve regurgitation and heart failure, and a history of two 2 previous aortic valve replacements, required a mitral valve replacement and right aorta-ventricular fistula repair. Intraoperatively, he lost 8 l of blood. However, rFVIIa given at the end of surgery reduced blood loss to 310 ml in the first hour post injection and to 3 ml 4 h post rFVIIa (fig. 5).

Laboratory Parameters

The patients had a mean of 18.5-fold increase in FVII levels measured 30 min after the injection of rFVIIa. Prothrombin time dropped by a mean of 12 s with rFVIIa treatment (fig. 6).

We concluded that a single perioperative dose of rFVIIa of 30 μg/kg was effective in achieving satisfactory haemostasis in these patients. No significant adverse events were reported.

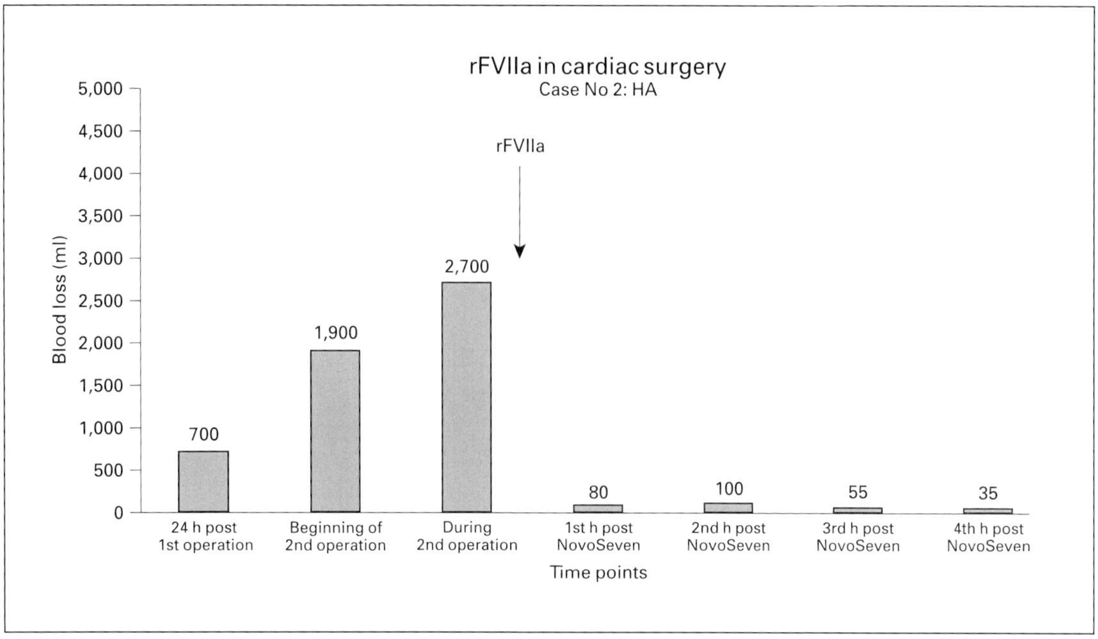

Fig. 2. rFIIa in cardiac surgery – case No. 2: HA: Reduction in blood loss by rFVIIa in a 73-year-old woman following mitral valve replacement and tricuspid valve repair [1].

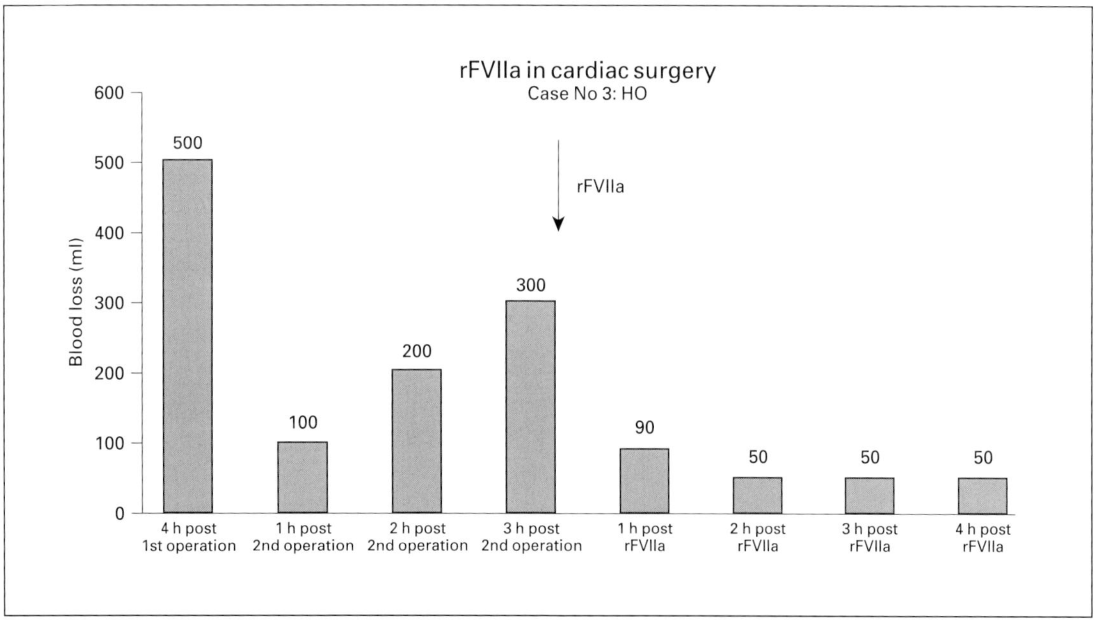

Fig. 3. rFVIIa in cardiac surgery – case No. 3: HO: Reduction in blood loss by rFVIIa in a 48-year-old woman following heart valve replacement surgery [1].

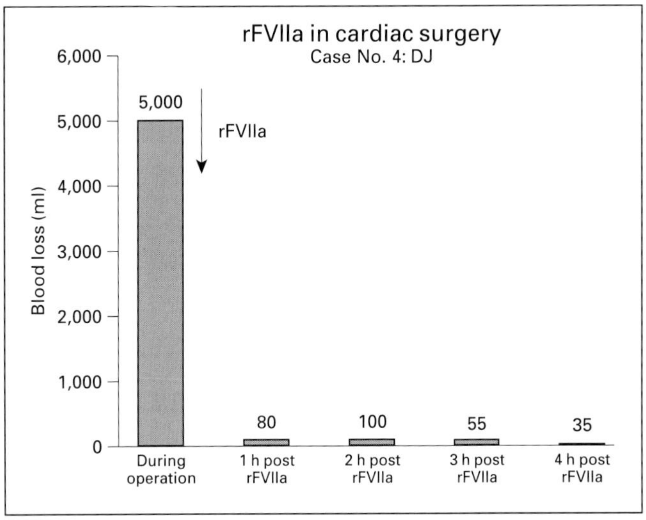

Fig. 4. rFVIIa in cardiac surgery – case No. 4: DJ: Reduction in blood loss by rFVIIa in a 65-year-old man following aortic valve repair [1].

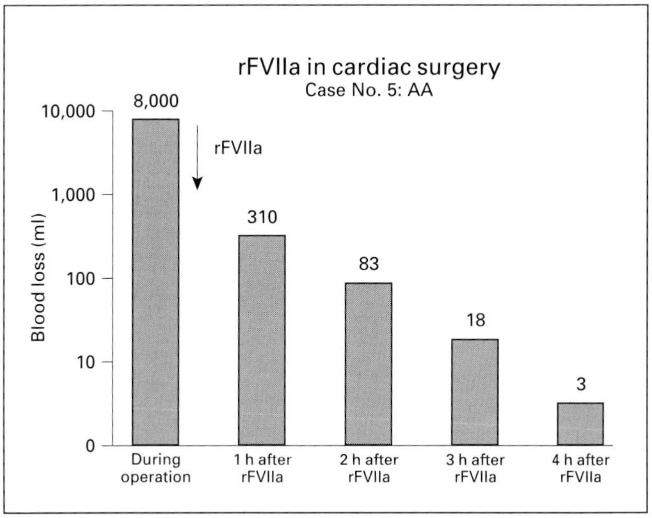

Fig. 5. rFVIIa in cardiac surgery – case No. 5: AA: Reduction in blood loss by rFVIIa in a 48-year-old man following mitral valve replacement and right aorta-ventricular fistula repair [1].

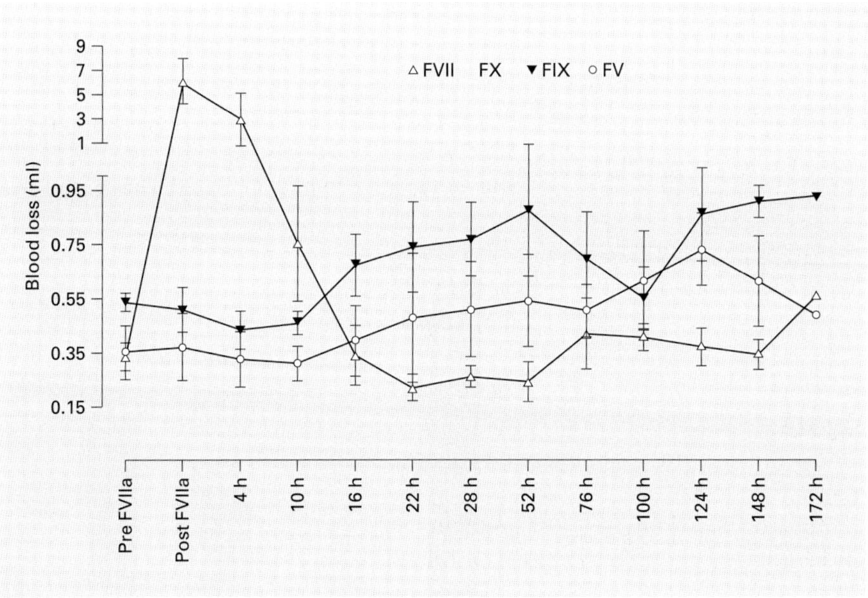

Fig. 6. Change in levels of FV, FVII, FIX and FX in patients 1–5 following administration of rFVIIa [1].

rFVIIa in Noncardiac Surgery

The medical literature contains several other reports on the use of rFVIIa outside the field of haemophilia. They include a report of 2 patients with Crohn's disease who suffered severe postsurgical intra-abdominal haemorrhage [2]. The patients, a 22-year-old woman and a 62-year-old man, presented with massive lower gastrointestinal bleeding requiring colectomy. Both patients had excessive postoperative abdominal haemorrhage, needing a large transfusion of blood components. As there was no resolution of the bleeding, they received rFVIIa in two doses each of 90 μg/kg. Their bleeding stopped immediately.

Two further cases of successful rFVIIa treatment for intractable surgical bleeding have been described by Laffan in 2000 [3]. A 20-year-old man with chronic myeloid leukaemia who suffered post-splenectomy haemorrhage, continued to bleed at a rate of 200 ml/h despite the use of haemostatic agents. He received rFVIIa, initially as a bolus of 90 μg/kg followed by infusion at 10 μg/kg/h for 18 h. His blood loss fell to 60 ml over 12 h. The second case was a 62-year-old woman with cervical carcinoma who had severe bleeding following anterior exenteration. Blood products were given to no avail but bleeding stopped when she received rFVIIa at 80 μg/kg followed by infusion of 10 μg/kg/h. Further cases in this centre are receiving bolus doses of rFVIIa without subsequent infusion.

In a report of peptic ulcer bleeding, a 59-year-old man with severe haematemesis and malaena had surgery to correct an ulcer in the duodenal bulb [4]. He required two further laparotomies due to bleeding and failed to respond to haemostatic agent. He received rFVIIa in a bolus dose of 90 μg/kg every 2 h for 21 h. The RBC transfusion requirement fell from more than 60 to 2 U over 16 h, allowing gastroduodenal artery embolisation to be performed.

A 70-year-old woman developed a large false aneurysm 20 days after thoracoabdominal aortic replacement [5]. A high dose of rFVIIa of 925 U/kg was infused into the aneurysm and a CT scan 2 months later showed complete occlusion of the aneurysm.

Promising results have also been seen with the use of rFVIIa as cover during prostatectomy [6]. In an ongoing randomised study, patients have received rFVIIa in a dose of 20 μg/kg or 40 μg/kg, or placebo. Results from 36 patients showed that blood transfusion was required in 60% of the placebo group compared with 38% of patients receiving the lower dose of rFVIIa and none of those receiving the higher dose.

Finally, rFVIIa has been used in an obstetric case with disseminated intravascular coagulation [8]. A 33-year-old woman with a twin pregnancy had continuous blood loss after Caesarean Section. Her bleeding was not resolved by a hysterectomy or a third laparotomy, but it did respond to rFVIIa at 90 μg/kg given in 9 doses 3 h apart.

rFVIIa in Trauma

Initial reports of the benefits of rFVIIa in trauma have included that of a 19-year-old Israeli soldier who had a bullet injury which severed the inferior vena cava [7]. Despite massive blood transfusion, he continued to bleed at a rate of 300 ml/min. Two doses of rFVIIa at 60 μg/kg, given 1 h apart, reduced bleeding to 10–15 ml/min.

This impressive result prompted a compassionate use study in Israel of rFVIIa in trauma and surgery [9]. Results are available from 4 trauma and 6 surgical patients with uncontrolled bleeding. Initial doses of rFVIIa were 60–120 μg/kg. All experienced a dramatic reduction in bleeding within 10–15 minutes of injection. A further publication by the same author reported 7 massively bleeding, multitransfused (median 40 U, range 25–49 U, of packed cells), coagulopathic trauma patients treated with rFVIIa (median 120 μg/kg, range 120–212 μg/kg) after failure of conventional measures. Administration of rFVIIa resulted in cessation of bleeding, with significant decrease of transfusion requirement to 2 U (range 1–2 U) [10].

Conclusion

Our data and other reported cases suggest that rFVIIa is effective and safe in controlling intractable surgical and traumatic bleeding. The effect is extremely rapid and may be seen in patients with normal coagulation profiles. However, rFVIIa regimes have varied and more research is needed to define its role as a universal haemostatic agent more clearly.

References

1 Aldouri M, Shafi T, Al Khudairi D, Al Bokhari E, Black L, Akinwale N, Osman Musa M, Al Homaidhi A, Al Fagih M, Borum Andreasen R: Effect of the administration of recombinant activated factor VII (rFVIIa; NovoSeven®) in the management of severe uncontrolled bleeding in patients undergoing heart valve replacement surgery. Blood Coagul Fibrinol 2000; 11(suppl 1):121–127.

2 White B, McHale J, Ravi N, Reynolds J, Stephens R, Moriarty J, Smith OP: Successful use of recombinant FVIIa (NovoSeven®) in the management of intractable post-surgical intra-abdominal haemorrhage. Br J Haematol 1999; 107:677–678.

3 Laffan MA, Cummins M: Recombinant factor VIIa for intractable surgical bleeding. 42nd annual meeting of American Society of Hematology, San Francisco, December 1–5, 2000, A4048 (abstract). Br J Am Soc Hematol 2000; 96;11:85b.

4 Vlot AJ, Mackaay AJC, Kramer MHH, Gaillard CAJM: Treatment of a severely bleeding patient without preexisting coagulopathy with activated recombinant factor VII. Am J Med 2000;108:421–422.

5 Liem KSAE, Biesma DH, Ernst SMPG, Schepens MAAM: Recombinant activated factor VII for false aneurysms in patients with normal haemostatic mechanisms. Thromb Haemost 1999;82:150–151.

6 Levi MM, Friederich PW, Heny CP, Messelink EJ, Breederveld D, Geerdink MGF, Spataro M, Kurth KH, Buller HR: Reduction in perioperative blood loss and transfusion requirements by NovoSeven® in patients undergoing transabdominal prostatectomy. Proceedings of the 6th Novo Nordisk symposium on the Treatment of Bleeding and Thrombotic Disorders. Copenhagen, May 3–4, 2001.

7 Kenet G, Walde R, Eldad A, Martinowitz: Treatment of traumatic bleeding with recombinant factor VIIa. Lancet 1999;354:1879.

8 Moscardo F, Perez F, De La Rubia J, Balerdi B, Lorenzo JI, Senent ML, Aznar I, Carceller S, Sanz MA: Successful treatment of severe intra-adominal bleeding associated with disseminated intravascular coagulation using recombinant activated factor VII. Br J Haematol 2001; 113:174–176.

9 Martinowitz U, Kenet G, Lubetzki A, Luboshitz J, Varon D: Recombinant activated factor VII (rFVIIa) for adjunctive hemorrhage control in trauma and surgery: The Israeli compassionate registry. Thrombosis and Haemostasis 2001;86(suppl):P2624 (abstract).

10 Martinowitz U, Kenet G, Segal E, Luboshitz J, Lubetsky A, Ingerslev J, Lynn M: Recombinant Activated Factor VII for Adjunctive Hemorrhage Control in Trauma. J Trauma (Injury, Infection and Critical Care) 2001;51:431–439.

Pathophysiology of Haemostasis and Thrombosis

Pathophysiol Haemost Thromb 2002;32(suppl 1):47–52

To General Haemostasis – the Evidence-Based Route

Elisabeth Erhardtsen

Novo Nordisk A/S, Bagsvaerd, Denmark

Key Words

Inhibitors · Thrombin · Safety · Traumata · Anticoagulant therapy · Impaired liver function

Abstract

Recombinant factor VIIa (rFVIIa) was developed for the treatment of bleeding in haemophilia patients with inhibitors and has also been used successfully in non-haemophilia patients with acquired antibodies against FVIII (acquired haemophilia). Based on dose-finding trials and a compassionate-use programme, rFVIIa was approved for use in haemophilia patients with inhibitors in 1996. At pharmacological doses, rFVIIa has been found to enhance thrombin generation on already activated platelets. Therefore, it is likely that rFVIIa will also be beneficial in providing haemostasis in other situations characterised by profuse bleedings and an impaired thrombin generation. Patients with thrombocytopenia have a decreased number of platelets and thus an impaired thrombin generation. A reduction in bleeding time was reported in approximately 50% of patients with thrombocytopenia and a prolonged bleeding time who participated in a trial of rFVIIa. Moreover, in 8 patients with 9 overt bleeds who were involved in the study, bleeding stopped in 7 episodes after rFVIIa administration. Case reports on the haemostatic effect of rFVIIa in thrombocytopenia have also been published. Reports have also been published on the successful use of rFVIIa in patients with platelet function deficiencies such as Glanzmann's thrombasthenia and Bernard-Soulier syndrome. A number of haemostatic changes occur after extensive trauma, surgery and bleeding, all of which potentially contribute to an impaired thrombin generation. The effect of rFVIIa has been demonstrated in a number of patients after trauma and bleeds and upper gastrointestinal bleeding episodes. Reports on the beneficial use of rFVIIa in liver transplantation have also been published. Several randomised blinded studies are now underway in e.g. hepatectomy, upper gastrointestinal bleedings, transplantations and intra-cerebral bleeds. In summary, rFVIIa may be an effective and safe method to induce haemostasis in patients within areas of coagulation factor deficiency or platelet disorders and the ongoing and planned randomised studies may lead the way to the use of rFVIIa in general haemostasis.

Introduction

Recombinant activated coagulation factor VII (rFVIIa) was developed for treatment of bleeding in haemophilia patients with inhibitors (HI) and has also been shown to be effective in the treatment of patients with acquired antibodies against FVIII (acquired haemophil-

KARGER

Fax + 41 61 306 12 34
E-Mail karger@karger.ch
www.karger.com

1424–8832/02/0327–0047$18.50/0

Accessible online at:
www.karger.com/journals/pht

Elisabeth Erhardtsen
International Medical Director Haemostasis
Novo Nordisk A/S, 53a Krogshojvej
DK–2880 Bagsvaerd (Denmark)
Tel. +45 4442 8888, Fax +45 4442 1213, E-Mail eer@novonordisk.com

ia). When administered in pharmacological doses rFVIIa enhances thrombin generation on the activated platelets. Patients with a variety of coagulation abnormalities characterized by uncontrollable bleedings and an impaired thrombin generation may benefit from rFVIIa in providing haemostasis. Clinical experience is available from a few patients with thrombocytopenia [1, 2] and other platelet defects and from patients with an impaired liver function [3, 4].

Clinical Experience with rFVIIa in Haemophilia Patients with Inhibitors

Administration of FVIII or FIX concentrates does not induce hemostasis in haemophilia patients who have developed inhibitors against FVIII or FIX as the factor concentrates are inhibited by the antibodies in the patient. rFVIIa has proven to be a safe and efficient agent for the treatment of bleeding episodes in HI patients and up to now, October 2001, more than 230,339 standard doses have been given.

Elective surgery has previously been contraindicated in HI patients who are at high risk of uncontrollable bleeding. However, major orthopaedic surgery such as hip or knee replacement has been successfully performed under the cover of rFVIIa in a number of HI patients [5–8]. The recommended dose was 90–120 μg/kg rFVIIa administered every 2 h during the first 24 h depending on the type of surgery and the clinical response. Furthermore, rFVIIa has been given in connection with minor surgery and dental surgery with success [8].

A prospective, double-blind, randomized trial comparing two doses of rFVIIa (35 and 90 μg/kg) in HI patients undergoing surgery was published in 1998 [9]. Bolus injections of rFVIIa were given every 2nd hour for the first 48 h and the same dose was then given every 2–6 h for an additional 3 days. Major surgical procedures such as synovectomies, hip arthroplasties, knee joint replacement were included. A statistically significant difference in efficacy favouring the high-dose group was observed from day 3 to day 5 with regard to maintained hemostasis, number of days of dosing required and in the number of injections. Based on the results from this study, the investigators concluded that rFVIIa appears to be an efficacious first-line agent in surgery in HI patients, and the 90 μg/kg dose was more effective for both minor and major procedures [9].

Since 1988 rFVIIa has been given in a compassionate use protocol to HI patients suffering from serious bleedings in whom all other therapies had failed. Essentially the same dose schedule as recommended in surgery was used. The overall effective response after 8 and 24 h in the first 55 consecutive bleeds was 91% and 90%, respectively [10].

84 patients were treated with two rFVIIa dosages (35 and 70 μg/kg) in a randomized, double-blind, multicentre trial including 179 joint, muscle, and mucocutaneous bleeding episodes [11]. A delay before start of treatment (8.4–10.0 h) may have contributed to the fact that there was no significant difference in efficacy between the two groups although a trend in both groups towards a better outcome for joint bleeds treated within 6 h was observed.

A home treatment study with rFVIIa was performed to optimize the treatment with rFVIIa in HI patients and make it more similar to that of haemophilia patients without inhibitors [12]. By using a dose of 90 μg/kg at 3-hour intervals in mild-to-moderate bleeding episodes an average of 2.3 doses were required to prevent the development of full joint or muscle bleeds [12].

Safety

In 664 patients (primarily HI patients) enrolled in Novo Nordisk-sponsored clinical trials, thrombotic events were reported in 4 HI patients and in 3 patients with acquired haemophilia (AH) (fig. 1).

An 8-year-old boy with HI developed signs of a left occipital infarct following a complicated course of subdural haematoma. A thrombotic complication related to the use of rFVIIa could not be excluded; however the investigator stated that an alternative explanation might have been ischemia due to pressure on the supplying vessel related to the mass effect of the haematoma.

A 4-year-old boy with HI developed a thrombosis in the right jugular vein two days following the insertion of a central venous catheter subsequent administration of rFVIIa.

A 36-year-old male with HI was treated initially with aPCC, and then with rFVIIa due to a large haematoma. Thirteen days later the patient experienced a massive gastrointestinal bleeding secondary to stress ulcer. The next day he developed abdominal pain, and a laparotomy revealed necrotic large bowel requiring resection, no evidence of thrombosis. The patient died nine days after surgery. The autopsy showed patent mesenteric vessels and a review of the colon pathology showed extensive gangrenous necrosis in several sections, but the mesenteric vessels were all patent.

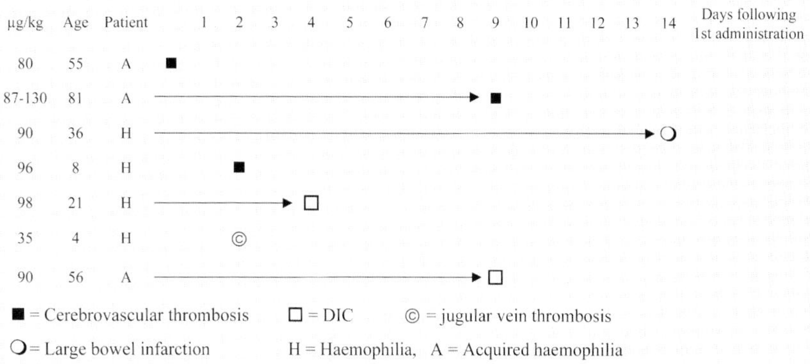

Fig. 1. Thrombotic complications reported in haemophilia trials.

A 21-year-old male with HI underwent extensive surgery twice for a large hip abscess. During the surgery extensive myonecrosis and necrotized fasciitis from knee to pelvis were noted. During the second surgery necessitated by extensive profuse bleeding, the patient experienced cardiac arrest refractory to resuscitation. An autopsy revealed microscopic microthrombi in the pulmonary vasculature.

The AH patients who were reported to have thrombotic events were multi-transfused patients. One, a 81-year-old male who was treated due to gastrointestinal bleeding had a DVT reported after infusion of porcine FVIII, human FVIII and rFVIIa. Another, a 55-year-old male who was treated for massive hepatic and subcapsular haemorrhage had an infarct reported after infusion of Feiba, Autoplex and rFVIIa. The third case was a 56-year-old female who had a lab DIC reported after infusion of blood transfusions and rFVIIa.

Recombinant FVIIa has been shown to induce hemostasis in severe HI patients both in major surgery [9], in serious bleedings in patients in whom all other therapies had failed [10], in joint and muscle bleeds [11], and in the home-treatment setting [12]. The complication of thrombotic events after treatment with rFVIIa seems to be rare and in most cases alternative aetiology was present (multi-transfusion, sepsis, etc.).

Recombinant FVIIa in Patients with an Impaired Thrombin Generation Other than Haemophilia

Patients with a decreased number of platelets have been shown to have a decreased thrombin formation [13]. In vitro studies have proven that the addition of rFVIIa in concentrations of 50–500 n*M* can cause a dose-dependent increase in the initial rate of thrombin generation and a shortening of the lag phase of platelet activation [14]. A study in 74 thrombocytopenic patients showed a shortening of the bleeding time in approximately 50% of the patients and in 8 thrombocytopenic patients rFVIIa had an effect on an open bleeding (nosebleed, vaginal bleed, oozing from catheters etc). The bleeding either stopped or slowed down (6/8 stopped; 2/8 slowed down) following administration of rFVIIa. Even in patients with a platelet count below 10,000 the bleeding stopped following the administration of 100 μg/kg of rFVIIa [15].

Furthermore, a case report on a hemostatic effect of rFVIIa in a thrombocytopenic patient has been published [16]. This patient had platelet counts below 5,000 indicating that rFVIIa has a hemostatic effect also in the presence of very low platelet counts.

Safety

No thrombotic events were reported in this population.

Preliminary studies including a few case reports indicate that rFVIIa may be of use in treating bleedings in patients with thrombocytopenia and platelet functional defects. Controlled trials are required for definitive proof of concept.

Severe Traumata Resulting in Profuse Bleeding

Other situations with a potential defective thrombin generation include patients who have been through severe traumata resulting in profuse bleeding requiring multiple transfusions of various blood products. Acute trauma in humans has been shown to initiate a number of hemostatic changes [13, 17]. A haemostatic effect has been demonstrated after administration of rFVIIa in a limited number of patients after trauma and bleedings [18–20].

The first patient with extensive bleedings following an intra-abdominal gunshot treated successfully with rFVIIa was published in 1999 [20]. This patient bled at a rate of 300 ml/min in spite of extensive transfusion therapy including packed red cells (5 l), fresh frozen plasma (3 l), platelets (20 units), cryoprecipitate (10 units) and antifibrinolytic therapy. In a desperate attempt to control the bleeding rFVIIa in a dose of 60 μg/kg was given leading to a decrease in rate of bleeding to 10–15 ml/min. Slow oozing from all wound surfaces continued, however, but stopped after a second dose of rFVIIa (60 μg/kg) given 1 h after the first one enabling surgical repair. The patient's condition remained stable, and no further blood loss occurred. Following this experience 9 more critically-ill, coagulopathic, multi-transfused trauma patients in whom conventional surgical and medical hemostatic treatment modalities had failed were treated with rFVIIa [19]. All patients suffered from uncontrolled bleeding despite surgical efforts and massive replacement therapy. Doses of rFVIIa were in the range of 40–120 μg/kg. Four of the patients received more than one dose (2–3). Blood requirements decreased considerably after rFVIIa. A median of 2 (range: 1–2.75) doses were required. Three patients expired – one suffered profound shock, hypothermia and acidosis for 14 h prior to administration of rFVIIa and died towards the end of surgery, two other patients died 4 weeks after treatment with rFVIIa from sepsis and liver failure related to the extensive liver hypoxia. Another case report on the successful use of rFVIIa in a woman experiencing heavy bleedings after stab wounds was published [18].

Safety

No thrombotic events were reported in any of the above mentioned patients.

The experience with rFVIIa in trauma patients experiencing excessive bleeding is based on case reports and indicates a hemostatic effect of rFVIIa administered in doses of 60–120 μg/kg. Controlled studies are needed to prove the beneficial effect of rFVIIa in these patients.

Defective Synthesis of FVII

A defect in the normal synthesis of FVII is reported in patients receiving oral anticoagulant therapy and in patients with impaired liver function.

Patients Receiving Oral Anticoagulant Therapy

FVII has been shown to be the earliest and the most sensitive of the coagulation factors to be affected by the oral anticoagulant therapy. Spontaneous haemorrhages represent a major treatment complication and have been reported to occur in around 10% of patients receiving oral anticoagulant therapy [21, 22]. These patients may also require reversal of their prolonged INR when invasive procedures are scheduled.

In a randomized, double-blind, placebo-controlled study, 28 healthy volunteers were administered acenocoumarol twice daily in order to boost INR values to within therapeutic levels. At INR values >2.0, levels of FVII were 4–17% [23]. Following the administration of one dose of rFVIIa ranged between 5 and 320 μg/kg the INR was normalized. Following doses of >120 μg/kg the INR remained normalized for 12 h. No signs of systemic activation of the coagulation system were seen.

One spontaneous nosebleed in a patient on warfarin with an INR of 2.9 has been reported successfully treated with two doses of 80 μg/kg rFVIIa [24]. Another report describes the use of rFVIIa in 7 adult patients who all had critically prolonged INR (range 3.2–13.9), 3 of whom required surgery. The doses administered ranged from 20 to 90 μg/kg and all patients were reported to have a positive outcome [25]. These observations indicate that rFVIIa may be used to reverse the effect of warfarin or other vitamin K antagonist therapy in cases where administration of vitamin K alone has been found insufficient. However, further studies are required to establish the optimal dose.

Patients with Impaired Liver Function

The liver is the principal site for synthesis and clearance of coagulation factors, components of the fibrinolytic system, and naturally occurring anticoagulants. The haematological abnormalities most frequently seen in cirrhotic patients include thrombocytopenia, a prolonged PT, and hyperfibrinolysis [26]. Cirrhotic patients do not generally experience bleeding episodes apart from upper GI bleeding but they are at an increased risk of bleeding from routine procedures such as liver biopsy, and also during major surgery such as liver transplantation [27].

Resulting from their complex coagulation pattern these patients may have an impaired thrombin generation and administration of rFVIIa in high doses may be able to compensate for the lack of the different coagulation parameters. A haemostatic effect has been proven in a limited number of liver disease patients [3, 4]. rFVIIa has also been evaluated in clinical trials with liver diseased patients. Ten cirrhotic patients whose PT did not correct to within 2 s above the control reference value were given three successive dosages of rFVIIa (5, 20, 80 μg/kg) during a 3-week period in a randomized study [28]. The PT transiently corrected to normal in all three dosage groups and the length of the effect was dose related.

A blind randomized study included 65 cirrhotic patients undergoing laparoscopic biopsy under the cover of rFVIIa in a dose range of 5–120 μg/kg [29]. Thirteen of the patients received a rescue dose of 80 μg/kg of rFVIIa. None required operative intervention or transfusion for blood loss after performing the biopsy and no clinically significant post-treatment changes in other coagulation parameters were observed. The authors concluded that the results suggest that laparoscopic liver biopsy can be performed safely and reliably using rFVIIa in patients in whom the standard procedure might be contraindicated due to coagulopathy.

Safety

Two thrombotic events were reported in the above mentioned patients. A 38-year-old male was undergoing laparoscopic liver biopsy. Six days after the administration of rFVIIa a routine Doppler ultrasound examination suggested thrombosis of the main portal vein. Eleven days after the administration of rFVIIa, the patient was admitted with peritoneal sepsis secondary to cirrhosis. The patient expired on day 13. The autopsy showed diffuse thrombosis of the portal vein system and massive alchemic hepatocellular necrosis. The microscopic examination revealed an overall pattern of acute thrombosis superimposed on pre-existing organizing thrombi.

A 43-year-old female with no prior history of liver disease was transferred to hepatology service with acute liver failure secondary to the use of Duract (bromfenac) for arthritis/club foot (approximately 5–6 months usage). The patient was treated with rFVIIa and subsequently underwent laparoscopic liver biopsy. Post-biopsy the patient's haematocrit dropped (from 34.3 to 28.5). The platelet counts also declined (from 129,000 to 119,000). No bleeding source was identified. No fibrinogen or PT values are available. The liver biopsy revealed 60–80% necrosis and the patient was referred to and successfully underwent liver transplantation.

Preliminary data seem to indicate that rFVIIa has effect in liver-diseased patients; however, controlled studies are required to prove the haemostatic effect and safety of rFVIIa in liver-diseased patients undergoing surgery or experiencing a spontaneous bleeding.

Building Strong Evidence

In vitro data conclude that rFVIIa can increase thrombin formation in different situations in which thrombin formation is insufficient. This is further substantiated by case stories and preliminary studies which indicate that rFVIIa may be able to control bleeding in different situations. A number of studies are under way in order to collect data from randomised placebo-controlled studies. These will focus on patients with liver disease undergoing surgery or experiencing spontaneous bleeding, patients with thrombocytopenia experiencing bleeding, patients with intracerebral haemorrhage, and patients with trauma.

Conclusion

Recombinant FVIIa is approved for treatment of haemophilia patients with inhibitors, and data on safety and efficacy of rFVIIa in the treatment of bleeding patients outside the haemophilia area are accumulating.

Acknowledgement

I thank Susan Eriksen for secretarial assistance.

References

1 Kristensen J, Killander A, Hippe E, Helleberg C, Ellegaard J, Holm M, Hedner U: Recombinant factor VIIa (rFVIIa) reduces the bleeding time in patients with thrombocytopenia. Abstract presented at the 35th Annual Meeting of ASH, St. Louis, December 3–7, 1993.
2 Poon MC, Demers C, Jobin F, Wu JWY: Recombinant factor VIIa is effective for bleeding and surgery in patients with Glanzmann thrombasthenia. Blood 1999;94:3951–3953.
3 Chuansumrit A, Treepongkaruna S, Phuapradit P: Successful invasive procedures in children with liver failure using recombinant factor VIIa. Haemophilia 2000;6:348.
4 Papatheodoridis GV, Chung S, Keshav S, Hardaker L, Pasi J, Burroughs AK: Recombinant factor VIIa is used in a Jehova's Witness with liver cirrhosis to correct prothrombin time, bleeding time, and thromboelastographic parameters, enabling safe percutaneous injection of hepatocellular carcinoma. Abstract presented at ISTH 1999.
5 Hedner U, Glazer S, Pingel K, Alberts KA, Blombäck M, Schulman S, Johnsson H: Successful use of recombinant factor Viia in patient with severe haemophilia A during synivectomy. Lancet 1988;ii:1193.
6 Hedner U, Ingerslev J: Clinical use of recombinant FVIIa (rFVIIa). Transfus Sci 1998;19: 163–176.
7 Ingerslev J, Freidman D, Gastineau D, Gilchrist G, Johnsson H, Lucas G, McPherson J, Preston E, Scheibel E, Shuman M: Major surgery in haemophilic patients with inhibitors using recombinant factor VIIa. Haemostasis 1996;26(suppl 1):118–123.
8 Lusher JM, Ingerslev J, Roberts HR, Hedner U: Clinical experience with recombinant factor VIIa. Blood Coagul Fibrinolysis 1998;9:119–128.
9 Shapiro AD, Gilchrist GS, Hoots WK, Cooper HA, Gastineau DA: Prospective, randomised trial of two doses of rFVIIa (NovoSeven) in haemophilia patients with inhibitors undergoing surgery. Thromb Haemost 1998;80:773–778.
10 Glazer S, Hedner U, Falch JF: Clinical update on the use of recombinant factor VII. Adv Exp Med Biol 1995;386:163–174.
11 Lusher JM, Roberts HR, Davignon G, Joist JH, Smith H, Shapiro A, Laurian Y, Kasper CK, Mannucci PM: A randomized, double-blind comparison of two dosage levels of recombinant factor VIIa in the treatment of joint, muscle and mucocutaneous haemorrhages in persons with haemophilia A and B, with and without inhibitors. rFVIIa Study Group. Haemophilia 1998;4:790–798.
12 Key NS, Aledort LM, Beardsley D, Cooper HA, Davignon G, Ewenstein BM, Gilchrist GS, Gill JC, Glader B, Hoots WK, Kisker CT, Lusher JM, Rosenfield CG, Shapiro AD, Smith H, Taft E: Home treatment of mild to moderate bleeding episodes using recombinant factor VIIa (NovoSeven) in haemophiliacs with inhibitors. Thromb Haemost 1998;80:912–918.
13 Hedner U, Erhardtsen E: Potential role for rFVIIa in transfusion medicine. Transfusion 2001;in press.
14 Kjalke M, Monroe DM, Hoffman M, Roberts HR, Hedner U, Ezban M: High-dose factor VIIa restores platelet activation and total thrombin generation in a model system mimicking hemophilia A or B conditions. Blood 1999;94(suppl 1):451a.
15 Kristensen J, Killander A, Hippe E, Helleberg C, Ellegaard J, Holm J, Kutti J, Mellqvist U-H, Johansson JE, Glazer S, Hedner U: Clinical Experience with recombinant factor VIIa in patients with thrombocytopenia. Haemostasis 1996;26(suppl 1):159–164.
16 Vidarsson B, Ônundarson P: Recombinant factor VIIa for bleeding in refractory thrombocytopenia. Thromb Haemost 2001;83:634–635.
17 Attar S, Boyd D, Layne E, McLaughlin J, Mansberger AR, Cowley RA: Alterations in coagulation and fibrinolytic mechanisms in acute trauma. J Trauma 1969;9:939–965.
18 Essex D, Bluth M, Gloster E, Dimaio T, O'Neill P, Waly D, Kurtz R, Strauss R: Successful use of recombinant factor VIIa (rFVIIa) for trauma-associated massive hemorrhage. Blood 2000;96:268a.
19 Martinowitz U, Kenet G, Onaca N, Luboshitz J, Amit J, Heim M: New treatment of uncontrolled hemorrhage in trauma/surgical patients: Induction of local hypercoagulation. Abstract presented at the 60th Annual Meeting of the American Association for the Surgery of Trauma, San Antonio, USA, October 2000.
20 Kenet G, Walden R, Eldad A, Martinowitz U: Tratment of traumatic bleeding with recombinant factor VIIa. Lancet 1999;354:1879.
21 Kearon C, Hirsh J: Management of anticoagulation before and after elective surgery. N Engl J Med 1997;336:1506–1511.
22 Gitter MJ, Jaeger TM, Petterson TM, Gersh BJ, Silverstein MD: Bleeding and thromboembolism during anticoagulant therapy: A population-based study in Rochester, Minnesota. Mayo Clin Proc 1995;70:725–733.
23 Erhardtsen E, Nony P, Dechavanne M, Ffrench P, Boissel JP, Hedner U: The effect of recombinant factor VIIa (NovoSeven(TM)) in healthy volunteers receiving acenocoumarol to an International Normalized Ratio above 2.0. Blood Coagul Fibrinolysis 1998;9:741–748.
24 Berntorp E, Stigendal L, Lethagen S, Olofsson L, Hedner U: NovoSeven (R) in warfarin-treated patients. Blood Coagul Fibrinolysis 2000;11:S113–S115.
25 Deveras RAE, Kessler CM: Recombinant factor VIIa (rFVIIa) successfully and rapidly corrects the excessively high international normalized ratios (INR) and prothrombin times induced by warfarin. Blood 2000;96:638a.
26 Paramo JA, Rocha E: Hemostasis in advanced liver disease. Semin Thromb Hemost 1993;19: 84–190.
27 Rapaport SI: Coagulation problems in liver disease. Blood Coagul Fibrinolysis 2000;11:S69–S74.
28 Bernstein DE, Jeffers L, Erhardtsen E, Reddy KR, Glazer S, Squiban P, Bech R, Hedner U, Schiff ER: Recombinant factor VIIa corrects prothrombin time in cirrhotic patients: A preliminary study. Gastroenterology 1997;113: 1930–1937.
29 Jeffers L, Balart L, Erhardtsen E, Chalasani N, Ortiz A, Pyrsopoulos N: Efficacy and safety of rFVIIa in patients with severe coagulopathy undergoing laparoscopic liver biopsy. Blood 1999;94(suppl 1):236a.

Pathophysiology of Haemostasis and Thrombosis

Author Index Vol. 32, Suppl. 1, 2002

Subject Index Vol. 32, Suppl. 1, 2002

KARGER
Fax +41 61 306 12 34
E-Mail karger@karger.ch
www.karger.com

Accessible online at:
www.karger.com/journals/pht

Extensive coverage of **thrombotic** and **hemorrhagic disease** and related **pathophysiology**

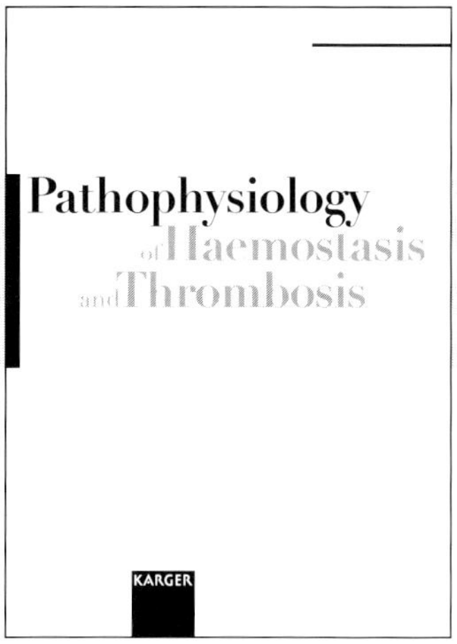

Pathophysiology of Haemostasis and Thrombosis

Title change

International Journal on Haemostasis and Thrombosis Research

Official Journal of the 'Mediterranean League against Thromboembolic Diseases'

formerly: Haemostasis

Senior Editor
H.C. Hemker, *Maastricht*

Managing Editor
J. Rosing, *Maastricht*

Associate Editors
G. Agnelli, *Perugia*
J.-J. Badimon, *New York, N.Y.*
S. Lévy-Toledano, *Paris*
J.-F. Schved, *Montpellier*

The journal 'Pathophysiology of Haemostasis and Thrombosis' publishes original papers in the field of thrombosis and haemostasis, a field whose importance for heart and vessel diseases is increasingly recognized. The last years have witnessed significant developments in the area, which are clearly reflected in the papers published here.
Original contributions report the latest findings on the pathology, physiology and biochemistry of hemorrhagic disease and thrombosis. In addition to in-depth studies of such topics as blood coagulation factors and fibrinolysis, readers will find extensive data on clinical results with heparin, oral anti-coagulation and newer anti-thrombotics. 'Pathophysiology of Haemostasis and Thrombosis' also provides practical information on the diagnosis and treatment of bleeding disorders and on fibrinolytic treatment. These experimental and clinical investigations are supported by occasional authoritative reviews to make the journal a full record of current research and its clinical implications.

Pathophysiology of Haemostasis and Thrombosis
2002: Volume 32
6 issues per volume
Language: English
ISSN 1424–8832
Listed in bibliographic services, including *Current Contents®, Index Medicus, Reference Update, Biological Abstracts, EMBASE/Excerpta Medica.*

Invitation for papers
Only original papers written in English will be considered.

Manuscripts should be sent to the Editorial Secretary:

T. Camphuisen-Engel
Universiteit Maastricht
Department of Biochemistry
Faculty of Medicine II, Level 4
PO Box 616
NL–6200 MD Maastricht (The Netherlands)

or one of the editors listed in the journal.

Selected contributions

Paroxysmal Nocturnal Hemoglobinuria and the Risk of Venous Thrombosis: Review and Recommendations for Management of the Pregnant and Nonpregnant Patient: ***Ray, J.G.*** *(Hamilton);* ***Burows, R.F.*** *(Clayton);* ***Ginsberg, J.S.*** *(Hamilton);* ***Burrows, E.A.*** *(Clayton)*

Influence of Fibrinogen Degradation Products on Thrombin Time, Activated Partial Thromboplastin Time and Prothrombin Time of Canine Plasma: ***Mischke, R.; Wolling, H.*** *(Hannover)*

Thrombolysis and Adjunctive Therapies in Acute Myocardial Infarction: ***Helft, G.*** *(Paris/New York, N.Y.);* ***Worthley, S.G.; Zaman, A.G.*** *(New York, N.Y.);* ***Samama, M.M.*** *(Paris);* ***Badimon, J.J.*** *(New York, N.Y.)*

Antithrombotic Activity of Orally Administered Low Molecular Weight Heparin (Logiparin) in a Rat Model: ***Hiebert, L.M.; Ping, T.; Wice, S.M.*** *(Saskatoon)*

Formation, Inhibition and Clearance of Plasmin in vivo: ***Chandler, W.L.*** *(Seattle, Wash.);* ***Alessi, M.C.; Aillaud, M.F.; Vague, P.; Juhan-Vague, I.*** *(Marseille)*

Intestinal Absorption of Low Molecular Weight Heparin in Animals and Human Subjects: ***Nissan, A.; Ziv, E.; Kidron, M.; Bar-On, H.; Friedman, G.; Hyam, E.*** *(Jerusalem);* ***Eldor, A.*** *(Tel Aviv)*

Personal rates per volume

Subscription	+ postage and handling	
CHF 439.–	+ CHF 28.80	Europe
CHF 439.–	+ CHF 42.70	Overseas
EUR 313.50	+ EUR 20.60	
USD 337.50	+ USD 28.80	

+ online subscription per volume:
CHF 39.– / EUR 28.– / USD 30.00

Institutional rates per volume

Subscription	+ postage and handling	
CHF 878.–	+ CHF 36.–	Europe
CHF 878.–	+ CHF 53.40	Overseas
EUR 627.–	+ EUR 25.80	
USD 675.00	+ USD 36.00	

+ online subscription per volume:
CHF 58.– / EUR 42.– / USD 45.00

Please enquire about reduced rates for members of the:
Dt. Arbeitsgemeinschaft für Blutgerinnungsforschung;
Int. Soc. of Hematology;
Med. League against Thromboembolic Diseases

Airmail surcharge per volume:
CHF 37.80 / USD 31.50

Prices subject to change
DEM price for Germany,
USD price for USA only

Read it online:
www.karger.com/journals/pht

Your gateway to full text, online reprints, forthcoming ToCs and our full line of publications.
Enjoy free access to abstracts, sample issues, and e-mail ToC-Alert service.

KARGER

KF 02066

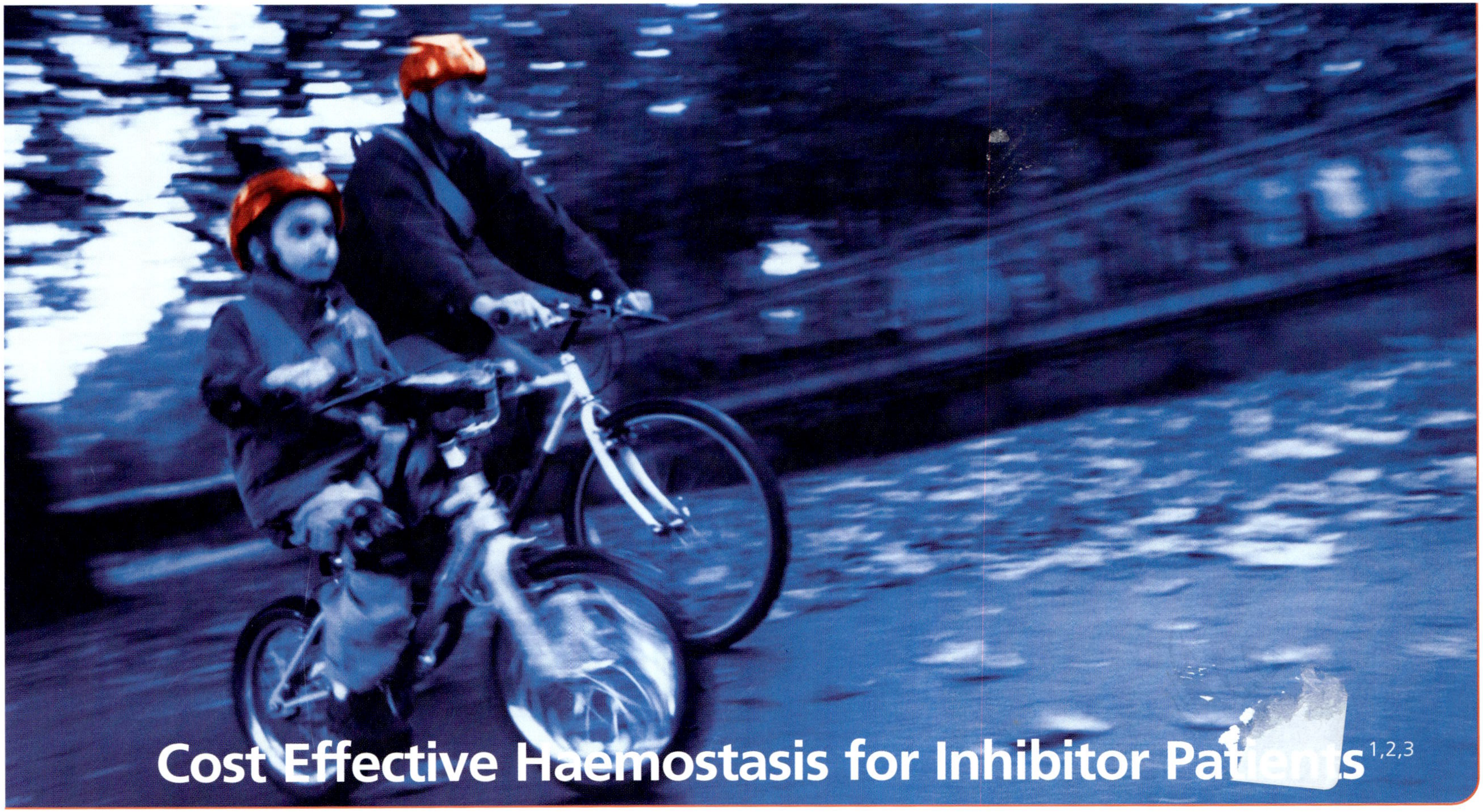

Cost Effective Haemostasis for Inhibitor Patients[1,2,3]

Presentation: Powder for injection with accompanying solvent for reconstitution (Water for Injections). Available in packs containing 60, 120 or 240 KIU rFVIIa. **Uses:** Bleeding episodes and surgery in patients with haemophilia with inhibitors to coagulation factors (FVIII or FIX) > 10 BU or in patients with antibody titre < 10 BU who are expected to have a high anamnestic response to FVIII or FIX. **Dosage:** The rFVIIa is dissolved in the accompanying solvent before use. After reconstitution the solution contains 30 KIU rFVIIa/ml (0.6 mg/ml). Administer by intravenous bolus injection; must not be mixed with infusion solutions or given in a drip. Initial dose of 4.5 KIU (90µg) per kg body weight, followed by administration in the dose range 3-6 KIU (60-120µg) per kg body weight depending on type and severity of haemorrhage or surgery performed. Inject over 2-5 minutes. For mild to moderate bleeding episodes in home-treatment setting: 1-3 doses at 3 hour intervals [4.5 KIU (90µg) per kg b.w.] to achieve haemostasis with additional dose to maintain haemostasis. Duration of home treatment should not exceed 24 hours. For serious bleeding episodes, initial dose 4.5 KIU (90 µg) per kg. b.w.; dose every two hours until clinical improvement. If continued therapy indicated, dosage interval can be increased successively. Major bleeding episode may be treated for 2-3 weeks or longer if clinically warranted. For surgery administer initial dose of 4.5 KIU (90µg) per kg. b.w. immediately before the procedure. Repeat dose at 2-3 hour intervals for first 24-48 hours. In major surgery continue dosing at 2-4 hour intervals for 6-7 days. Dosage interval may then be increased to 6-8 hours for further 2 weeks. Treatment may be up to 2-3 weeks until healing has occurred. **Contra-indications:** Known hypersensitivity to mouse, hamster or bovine protein. **Precautions:** NovoSeven should only be administered in centres specialised in the treatment of patients with coagulation factor VIII or IX inhibitors. Home treatment should be in close collaboration with a haemophilia centre. Possibility of thrombogenesis or induction of DIC in conditions in which tissue factor could be expected in circulating blood, e.g. advanced atherosclerotic disease, crush injury, septicaemia, or DIC, and surgery with major tissue destruction. Since NovoSeven contains trace amounts of mouse, bovine and hamster proteins there is a remote possibility of the development of hypersensitivity. Avoid simultaneous use of prothrombin complex concentrates, activated or not. **Use in pregnancy:** Only administer to pregnant women if clearly needed. Not known if excreted in human milk; exercise caution when administering NovoSeven to nursing women. **Side Effects:** Most frequently reported non-serious adverse reactions: haemorrhage, rash, fever. Serious adverse reactions: arterial thrombotic events (such as myocardial infarction or ischaemia, cerebrovascular disorders and bowel infarction); venous thrombotic events (such as pulmonary embolism and thrombophlebitis) and haemorrhage. For the thrombotic events all patients were predisposed and in the reported haemorrhages NovoSeven was not administered in accordance with the recommended dosage regimen. Coagulation abnormalities including low platelet count, low fibrinogen and presence of FDP and D-dimer have been reported from clinical trials. Two FVII-deficient patients have developed antibodies against FVII after treatment with NovoSeven. One patient, with a history of allergic reactions to several other drugs, experienced an anaphylactic reaction after receiving NovoSeven. Patients predisposed to thrombotic disorders or DIC and patients with a history of allergic reaction should be carefully monitored during therapy with NovoSeven. **Marketing Authorisation numbers:** NovoSeven 60 KIU EU/1/96/006/001; NovoSeven 120 KIU EU/1/96/006/002; NovoSeven 240 KIU EU/1/96/006/003. **Legal Category:** POM. **Basic NHS Price:** NovoSeven 60 KIU (1.2 mg) £705.00; NovoSeven 120 KIU (2.4 mg) £1410.00; NovoSeven 240 KIU (4.8 mg) £2820.00. **Further information:** Full prescribing information can be obtained from: **Novo Nordisk Limited**, Broadfield Park, Brighton Road, Crawley, West Sussex RH11 9RT. Tel: 01293 613555 Fax: 01293 613535. **Date of preparation:** February 2002. N7/FBI/030.

novo nordisk®

1. Stewart A J et al. Blood Coagulation and Fibrinolysis 1998;9 (Suppl 1): S93 - S95. 2. Odeyemi IAO and Guest JF. Abstract presented at the 6th Novo Nordisk Symposium on Treatment of Bleeding and Thrombotic Disorders, May 2001. 3. Odeyemi IAO and Guest JF. Poster presented at the Annual Meeting of The American Society of Haematology, San Francisco, USA, December 2000

* In haemophilia patients with inhibitors. Lusher JM et al. Haemophilia 1998;4: 790-798. A randomised, double-blind comparison of two dosage levels of recombinant factor VIIa in the treatments of joint, muscle and mucotaneous haemorrhages in persons with haemophilia A and B, with and without inhibitors.

NovoSeven®
Eptacog alfa (activated)

*Effective Haemostasis in Critical Bleeding**

F 02018